What experts **TIME TO LISTEN:**

Dr. Rynearson's book *Time to Listen* highlights the challenges American medicine has faced when the financial reward is more for doing procedures than for what the patient needs–someone to listen. As the debate on health-system reform continues, the value of listening should be recognized and paid for. I highly recommend reading this book in order to better understand how mental health plays such an important role in physical health and needs to be an important component of health system reform.

— *J. James Rohack, M.D.*
Director, Scott & White Center for Healthcare Policy
Temple, Texas

Robert Rynearson, M.D., is a nationally renowned psychiatrist, clinician, and teacher who has taken his experience with patients and distilled his hard-earned knowledge of the art of psychotherapy into this wonderfully rich volume. Filled with clinical vignettes and creative approaches to treatment, the book is a fascinating read as well as a lesson to all clinicians on how to approach the psychotherapeutic enterprise with flexibility and to adapt techniques derived from psychotherapy research in many areas such as the use of art, hypnosis, facial asymmetry, psychoanalysis, and analytic psychotherapy.

For beginners and experienced clinicians alike, this book has the additional value of a professional memoir by a caring, empathetic psychiatrist who merges treatment and humanism in a profoundly moving fashion.

— *Arthur T. Meyerson, M.D.*
Clinical Professor of Psychiatry
New York University School of Medicine

This is an important book about resolving inner conflicts, restoring our vitality, and reviving our capacity for meaningful relationships. It is entertaining, insightful, relevant, and useful.

— Bill Reed, M.D.
General Internist
Chicago, Illinois

TIME TO LISTEN

TIME TO LISTEN

Robert R. Rynearson, M.D.

Anabeth Hill

Best wishes

Bob   6/26/10

INK BRUSH PRESS

Library of Congress Control Number:
009934076
ISBN 978-0-9824405-3-7
© Robert R. Rynearson, M.D., 2010
All Rights Reserved
Manufactured in the United States
Published by Ink Brush Press, Temple, Texa

Art on cover: from a painting by one of Dr. Rynearson's patients who worked in art therapy to overcome the mania he suffered from being bipolar.

Cover Design by Lisa Craig.

With all my love, I dedicate this book to Marjie.

. . . it is the disease of not listening . . . that I am troubled withal.

William Shakespeare

Contents

Acknowledgments

I'm grateful to the many people who helped me with this book Sandy Sheehy, editor and published author, edited the first round of my ramblings. Marjie Rynearson, story structure expert, then gave it some order, and Carroll Wilson with his expert editing turned it into a real book. Others were also generous with their help: Ed Rynearson, Jim Rynearson, Karen Snyder, Katherine Rynearson Tagemeier, Kimberly Rynearson, Kali Rynearson, Mary Hutchings Reed, Bill Reed, Barbara Burges, Suzie Isaacs, Deborah Haude, Arlene Hirsch, and Ivan Dee. Additional thanks go to our friends Beryl Lawn, Dian Ruud, Steve Lemmons, Gary Hansen, Arthur Meyerson, M.D., Forrest Gist, Carol Bernstein, M.D., Paul Ekman, Ph.D., Sue Goldstein and Sherry Craven.

Thanks also to the professionals with whom I worked over the years and to the many patients from whom I learned so much. To ensure confidentiality, I have changed the names of patients mentioned in this book.

Introduction

This book has a great title—*Time to Listen*—but in some ways it is a misleading one. That's because Bob Rynearson, Ryno as he's known to all his friends, family, and colleagues, is more than a listener; he is also a watcher, a thinker, a boundary breaker, a physician, a healer, and an artist. You learn about all these facets of this well-rounded man, in the stories he tells, the fascinating examples of how he, indeed, takes time not only to listen, but also to watch and to encourage with innovative therapy.

Early in the book you learn how Ryno sensed that the time required for conventional psychodynamic psychotherapy was becoming a luxury which would no longer be affordable. I strongly suspect that even without that incentive, Ryno would have sought a quicker, more direct way to help his patients. He is an impatiently patient man; he wants to get to the heart of the matter, not to linger on the side roads, but get to what he calls "the superhighway to repressed emotions." As a lifelong student of emotion, I was delighted to find a psychiatrist who also focused on the emotions that patients feel strongly without knowing the source or nature of those feelings and that Ryno was willing to use many different methods to achieve "the superhighway to insight."

Early in his career his own interest and talent as an artist led him to use art and poetry to help his patients confront their feelings and allow him to better understand them. In addition to art Ryno used other innovative techniques, among them two new methods for getting on that superhighway: Profile Self-Confrontation and the Relived Emotional Status Exam. Profile Self-Confrontation (PSC) allows the patient and therapist to see two views of the patient's face at once, captured by two video cameras, one showing the left side and the other the right side of the face and to watch how each side of the face is markedly different.

Ryno tells how Werner Wolff, a nearly forgotten early Gestalt psychologist, explored the difference in the messages signaled by the left side and right side of the face with still photographs. I met Wolff near the end of his life and the beginning of mine. He was one of many German Jewish refugees from Nazi Germany, and he was teaching at Bard College. In 1955 I was twenty-one years old and a first-year graduate student in clinical psychology. I became interested in what was then called "nonverbal behavior" and searching the literature, I found Wolff's book on expressive behavior that had been written some fifteen years earlier. Among many other fascinating observations and experiments, Wolff described his findings and showed some illustrations of the differences between the two sides of the face.

Ten years later, equipped with a Ph.D. and my first grant from the National Institute of Mental Health, I studied still photographs of both sides of patients' faces when they first entered a mental hospital and then again when they had recovered from a severe episode. A year's work revealed nothing consistent in the patients' profiles or in the difference in the two sides of faces revealed in the still photographs.

Did I fail because I was using still photographs and not the motion that video provides, which is what Ryno uses in PSC? Or was it because in the middle sixties I had only a very rough, crude method for measuring what the left and right sides conveyed? It was not until nearly fifteen years later that I developed the precise facial measurement tool called the Facial Action Coding System (FACS) but regrettably, I never returned to those patient photographs using FACS.

I was by then studying other matters.

A third reason I failed may have been that I was not asking the patients to explore their feelings as they were being videotaped in order to watch their own expressions on each side of their faces. I have seen some of Ryno's videos and they are dramatic. He is a very gifted clinician. He is totally focused on his subjects when he talk with them. The crucial element may well be the relationship—the listening, watching, intuitive, sensitive doctor who is talking with the patient during this process. I hope this book will serve to stimulate some scientists to do research using the PSC technique.

The Relived Emotional Status Exam described in the book and provided in the appendix is a slight modification of a tool I invented to allow subjects to re-experience emotions in the laboratory where we could measure precisely their facial expressions and their autonomic nervous-system activity (heart rate, blood pressure, respiration, sweating, etc.). At first I feared that when research subjects were in a laboratory with wires attached to their bodies, they would find it very hard to reexperience past emotions. Not the case. I soon learned that nearly everybody has a story he or she wants to tell about an intense experience of emotions that all humans feel, albeit often in different ways with different consequences. Just give patients the invitation to relive a strong emotional experience such as anger, fear, disgust, etc., and for most people, healing begins to register immediately. This exam, coupled with PSC, has proven to be invaluable.

Hearing about this research, Ryno immediately sensed how this could be of benefit in helping patients with emotions that are repressed, in their getting in touch with these emotions, and in finding that superhighway to insight. And indeed, it has been helpful as Ryno explains in his book.

Time To Listen will be useful and interesting to anyone in the healing professions, not just psychiatry, and to people who want to better understand themselves. It is also a book for psychotherapists, whether they are psychiatrists, psychologists, social workers, or ministerial counselors. I hope this book with its actual case histories or "life stories" will stimulate other research clinicians to not only use Profile Self-Confrontation and listening skills, but to do research on the benefits of such therapy.

I can't close without describing Ryno the man, how we met, and what our friendship has meant to me. It must be at least thirty years ago, probably closer to forty, when he invited me to give a lecture at Scott & White Hospital in Temple, Texas, where he chaired the psychiatry department. He is a large man, almost a giant, slim, intense, open, and engaging, and soon we became personal friends. He is the older brother I never had, *sans* the sibling rivalry that so often is natural among male siblings. Despite the distance between where we live, we have managed to sustain a loving friendship. It is a privilege to know this man. I am glad he is inviting readers to become acquainted with him through this compelling book.

By Paul Ekman, Ph.D.
Professor Emeritus of Psychology
University of California, San Francisco

Preface

A man who listens speaks to eternity.
Proverbs 21:28

When one of my patients experiences an important insight, the patient and I are one. It is a magical moment, and for me that's the whole thing. I believe that life is meant to hold magic for us all. The challenge is knowing how to achieve that moment with my patients. How do we get there? How do we combine the art of healing with the science of medicine?

I cannot overstate the effectiveness of compassionate listening. Before sophisticated diagnostic tests were developed, therapists had to listen. These days we must, if we wish to be genuinely effective, continue taking the time to listen. I find that if I listen long enough, listen until I truly hear, I am usually able to determine the real cause of a patient's symptoms. Most simply need compassionate listening. I strive to make listening into an active process: I ask questions to encourage a patient to speak, then remain silent, listening, until another question seems necessary. I might ask "How long have you had this problem? What does your problem keep you from doing? Tell me more. What medicines are you taking? What have medical doctors told you?" My list of questions is a long one, and there are new ones that come up in nearly every case.

The important thing is to ask enough questions to get a patient talking, then for me to stop talking, to listen. In seeking that magical moment when a patient breaks through into meaningful insight, my driving force is listening, and my greatest tool is compassion. I'm never satisfied with making a snap decision based upon immediate evidence and prescribing a pill. It is important to limit the amount of medicine and the number of procedures, for they can be intrusive, expensive, ineffective, and sometimes dangerous.

Socrates in his trial for heresy urged people to look closely at themselves. "The unexamined life," he declared, "is not worth living." After 2500 years, his advice is as vital as ever. All of us can and should maximize our energy for living, for doing the work that will provide us with a good measure of bliss, security, intimacy, and loving relationships so ultimately we can affirm ours were lives worth living.

To make a positive difference in the lives of others I must help create a safe environment for them to speak. Most important of all I must be fully present and open during the necessary and crucial time to listen.

Chapter One
Artist or Physician?

By the age of seventeen, I had looked at myself in the bathroom mirror in our Rochester, Minnesota, home thousands of times. But that summer of my seventeenth year I learned the crucial difference between looking at something and actually seeing what's there.

That moment of revelation became a turning point that literally changed my life, and the revelation itself became a touchstone for all that followed. In 1950 I graduated from Rochester High School, a lanky, uncertain boy-man who by that time had earned the rank of Eagle Scout, earned my own money as a golf caddy, and earned a perhaps-deserved reputation for hubris. But also by 1950 I had suffered through a deep depression, and at that point in my young life I was preparing with great dread and trepidation to go forward on a path established in loyalty to my father and in direct opposition to what I knew was right and best for me.

The jolting revelation occurred serendipitously, within the walls of O'Connor's Men's Store, the finest haberdasher in Rochester. I had been accepted into the Harvard Class of 1954, and naturally I would require a wardrobe appropriate for the Ivy League. My father was an endocrinologist at the Mayo Clinic in Rochester, and he nodded in approval as I tried on various garments the afternoon before I left for Boston. With the help of an attentive sales clerk we found something suitable on the rack—a substantial blue pinstripe suit with natty cuffed pants, but as I pulled on the suit coat in front of a mirror that allowed a view from three different angles, I caught sight of the left side of my face. I was stunned. It looked weak and profoundly sad.

For an instant I thought, "That can't be me." I'd thought of myself as confident, smart, and outgoing. I might even have been perceived by others as arrogant. Now, confronted with my left profile, I felt sick to my stomach. I turned quickly to my right profile, which was more reassuring, more comfortable for me.

My father said, "I've heard that movie actors only allow the

1

camera to shoot their 'good side.' Everybody has a side they don't like." The repulsion I felt for my left side I now know was disgust about the unconscious feelings I was trying to hide, feelings that showed on the left side of my face. I figured out later that the left profile I saw during my fitting at O'Connor's reflected a deep conflict. I had until that moment been unable to recognize much less deal with that conflict.

Just the year before I had confessed to my mother that I hoped I would catch tuberculosis so I could go stay at a TB sanitarium for two or three years. What I knew of these treatment centers made them seem appealing because they were often in scenic locations with plenty of fresh air and a lot of gentle nurturing. The pharmaceutical cure for tuberculosis was still in the future. I had imagined the sanitarium as a refuge, a sanctuary where I'd be wrapped in blankets and hand-fed by kind nurses. I suppose I thought it would be a place where I could escape my then overwhelming emotional bind.

My father, known by his friends and colleagues as "The Great Healer," prided himself on never having urged me to become a doctor. Even so, I was sure he desperately wanted me to follow in his professional footsteps. My mother, on the other hand, was a frustrated musician. Her father had been an accomplished pianist, so talented that he was asked to accompany Enrico Caruso when the famous opera singer gave a recital in Pittsburgh, Pennsylvania. My mother had inherited her father's gift, but guided by the sanctions placed on well-bred young women in the first decade of the twentieth century, he refused to send her to college or to a music conservatory. She played the piano at home but not in public. She wanted me to realize her own dreams by becoming a musician, a writer, or some other kind of artist. Unlike my dad she made her ambitions for me explicit, constantly urging me to go out and experience things and write them down in a journal. I knew in my gut that there was no way I could satisfy both my parents.

My parents' conflicting expectations created a struggle I could not deal with at that time, so I internalized or repressed it. When I internalized this struggle, it manifested itself in an irrational

2

desire for an isolating illness, tuberculosis. I believe it was also responsible for the sadness that my left profile had exposed as I looked in O'Connor's three-part mirror.

If I could have developed tuberculosis on my own, it would have been a prime example of letting physical illness provide a way out of an intolerable emotional bind. Although concerned about my fantasy, my mother didn't send me to a psychiatrist. The Mayo Clinic was world-renowned for state-of-the art care, but at that time it had only one psychiatrist, and he specialized in adults.

I endured my situation more or less passively. With my new suit from O'Connor's folded in my trunk, I went off to Harvard. Although no one wrapped me in blankets and hand-fed me in Cambridge, I felt a geographic advantage. It was more than a thousand miles from Rochester, and I soon stopped fantasizing about developing tuberculosis. For four years I focused effectively on my studies, but when I entered the University of Minnesota Medical School the fall after my graduation from Harvard, I found myself feeling surprised and totally out of place. "How did I get here?" I wondered.

Some of my professors wondered why I was there as well. At the end of my freshman year in medical school my class size was reduced by fifty percent. I was still hanging on, but to the very bottom rung of the students who remained, and the dean informed me that I would not be welcome back for my second year. Given my strong grades at Harvard and in my pre-med summer courses, my professors couldn't believe that I had not done better. The dean called me to his dean's committee meeting and asked if I was having trouble with women or alcohol. Was I studying hard enough?

Finally, my physiology professor Maurice Vischer posed a possible explanation: "Since your father is a Mayo Clinic physician, perhaps you are ambivalent about becoming a doctor. Maybe you are failing in order to hurt him." His suggestion took my breath away.

"Yes!" I said, experiencing a rush of relief. For the first time in years I cried. At that instant my inner conflict dissolved, and I

3

experienced the frisson, the shudder of emotion, the thrill of transcending that conflict and finding unity within myself. Now I had insight. He suggested I see a psychiatrist but I replied, "I don't think I need to see a psychiatrist. I think I need to decide whether I want to be a doctor or hurt my father, because the way I'm going, I'm only hurting myself."

Although I did not see a psychiatrist, the dean's committee allowed me to continue. Over the ensuing years I experienced a meteoric rise in class standing, even as I wrestled with the issue of whether I really wanted to become a physician. Along with struggling with that question, of course, I faced having to decide exactly what sort of physician to become from the dozens of possible specialties. Between my third and fourth years in medical school, I reluctantly accepted a two-month elective position in psychiatry at Mayo. And it was, to say the least, a life-changing experience. There I saw miraculous things happen that I did not understand. I saw dysfunctional people become functional without medication, without surgery, and sometimes without even words. To me psychiatry was an intriguing mystery, and I decided during that summer at Mayo to continue my medical career as a doctor trying to better understand how life stresses affect people's functioning.

I had decided to become a doctor, which would please my father, but I had chosen psychiatry as a specialty, which would not please him at all. I waited to break the news until a weekend in October when we were duck hunting. Sitting in a blind on a slough off the Mississippi River, I turned to him and said, "Dad, I've decided to become a psychiatrist."

He said, "I thought you were going to be a real doctor." But I knew then, in my mid-twenties that being a psychiatrist was being a "real doctor," and my professional experience in subsequent decades supported this conviction. Instead of agonizing all my life over the conflict between being an artist to please my mother and a doctor to please my father, I finally gained insight into what was causing my distress. If they were alive I am sure they would both be pleased that I became a psychiatrist who depended heavily on the creative process to help patients and to help myself.

4

After five decades of treating psychiatric patients and teaching medical students and residents, I remain convinced that treatment is most successful for many emotional ailments and most physical complaints when both the therapist and the patient understand insights which come from confronting repressed conflicts face-to-face, as opposed to merely approaching the conflicts intellectually. It is the difference between being able to point to Paris on a map and reliving your own experiences of walking the Champs Elysees on an April morning.

For example, let's imagine that a man who has been in analysis for six years because he cannot maintain lasting relationships with women may confide to a friend that his failure is due to his mother's emotional inconsistency—warm one day, rejecting the next. He understands that intellectually, so he is confident that his impending fifth marriage will endure. The much-divorced fellow could be accurate and yet wrong. Experience has taught me that unless this man could find a therapist who would get him to *relive* feeling the pain of those repressed encounters, his next marriage would follow the same path as the previous four.

After I graduated from medical school in 1958, Marjie and I and our one-month-old son drove our 1952 green Plymouth across the country to Seattle. As I was driving I grew more unsettled about how little I knew about medicine, and I had increasing doubts about being a doctor. "Name the cranial nerves," I said to myself. I remembered my mnemonic helper, which was "On Old Olympus's Towering Top, a Finn and German Viewed Some Hops." Good, I told myself, but what did V stand for? Vegus. Okay. How about the mnemonic for the wrist bones? "Never Lower Tillie's Pants, Grandma May Come Home." What does the L stand for? Lunate. Moon-shaped. Right. I had developed innovative mnemonics for everything. My pretest anxiety had always been whether I could remember my mnemonics. Now my pre-internship anxiety was whether remembering such mnemonics had anything to do with being a doctor.

When we arrived in Seattle, we moved into an apartment just across the street from the Virginia Mason Clinic and Hospital. I had a rotating internship and was assigned to medicine, surgery, obstetrics, gynecology, pediatrics, and the emergency room. I was to be on call every other night and every other weekend, starting my rotation on the medicine service. Being six feet seven inches tall, I had designed my own internship uniform complete with big pockets and holders for the required tuning fork and reflex hammer. I wore white bucks with red soles and jingled when I walked. I must most certainly have looked doctorly. On my first day on the medicine service, I was told to cover all medicine problems for six hospital floors. I was terrified. So, I went to the sixth floor of the hospital, strode up to the nurses' station in my strange outfit, knocked loudly on the desk, and demanded to see the head nurse. She came out and asked me what I wanted. She was in her fifties and was scowling. "I just want to introduce myself," I said. "I'm Dr. Rynearson, and I want to get one thing straight."

She arched her eyebrows and said, "And what is that, Dr. Rynearson?"

I replied, "You, Mrs. Nordstrom, are the boss. I don't know anything, and I will need all the help you can give me." She smiled and held out her hand. I said the same thing to the nurse in charge on all six floors.

Later that day, Mrs. Nordstrom called, saying a patient in Room 611 was coughing up blood. I knew the technical term, but I had no idea what to do about it. She gave me the following instructions:

First, go to the room and introduce yourself and shake his hand. All patients need touching. Then sit down and ask him how he is feeling. You know, anyone who is coughing up blood must be very frightened. Then look at the spots of blood on his tissue. Talk about any other medical problems he has, then begin your physical, listening carefully to his chest. And tell him you are going to call your staff doctor, Dr. Morgan, who is an expert in lung problems. Then come back to the nursing station, call Dr. Morgan, and describe your evaluation.

Dr. Morgan, who had been trained at Mayo, came in and told me I had done a good job and taught me how to diagnose and treat a patient with hemoptysis (expectoration of blood). When we got back to the nurses station, he told me the tests I should order. As I gave the chart to Mrs. Nordstrom, I shook her hand and thanked her for helping me learn how to be a doctor.

After the internship in Seattle, Marjie and I went back to Mayo for a three-year psychiatric residency. When I had completed four months, Marjie, in her last trimester of pregnancy had an obstetric complication called placenta previa, and we rushed her to the hospital where she was transfused and placed flat in bed for five weeks. Once the baby was born, my mentor, Dr. Howard Rome, said he would help us find a three-month rotation where Marjie could recuperate in the sun.

Dr. Rome contacted Dr. Edwin Weinstein in Charlotte Amalia in the U.S. Virgin Islands and arranged for me to take a three-month elective with his supervision. We were to start working together on January 1, 1960. But just after Christmas I got a call that Dr. Weinstein had resigned, and much to my surprise the medical director offered the job to me at Dr. Weinstein's salary. To say it was a learning experience would be a magnificent understatement. Upon arrival I found I was in charge of terribly disturbed inpatients in a closed psychiatric unit at the Knud Hansen Government Hospital, evaluating psychiatric outpatients, and consulting with school districts in St. Croix and St. John's about their children with mental problems.

In dealing with all this stress I became increasingly anxious, but I couldn't seem to realize what was wrong with me. The anxiety manifested itself as an overwhelming fear of "mahogany birds," huge flying cockroaches. When I returned home each evening, I told Marjie to shut all windows and doors because I was terrified that the "mahogany birds" would invade our house. Marjie could not understand my irrational behavior, and thankfully, as time went on, my anxiety diminished and my phobia disappeared.

Before this, the only exposure I'd had to psychiatry was on the hospital inpatient unit at Mayo where I had started out observing group therapy, so that's how I began at Knud Hansen Hospital.

Group therapy in an enclosed outdoor area began at eight o'clock every morning. The first morning I told patients and staff that we would be absolutely free and open to discuss any problems. After a long silence, one of the women patients asked if they could say absolutely anything they wanted to within the group. I said "Yes, absolutely." After another long silence, a female patient asked again, "We can say anything? We won't be punished?" I reassured her that she could talk about anything that troubled her. She paused briefly, pointed her finger at an aide, and said in an angry voice, "Get the hell out of here! You have broken into my room twice and made me suck your cock."

Two other women spoke out: "And you raped us." At this point, everyone looked at the aide. He was so frightened he jumped up, ran to the wall of the enclosure, and climbed over. We never saw him again. These women patients had been enduring abuse because they were too afraid to speak up. By empathetic listening, I had given them permission to speak out and in doing so, they had taken the power the aide had over them away from him and claimed it for themselves.

My residency training had been superb in the Mayo Clinic Psychiatric Department where I learned much more than any text could teach. We were expected to challenge our instructors, which was a welcome way to grow in the profession. I recall, for example, that in my first year in 1959 I was assigned to conduct psychoanalytic treatment of a homosexual. At that time homosexuality was categorized as a mental illness by the American Psychiatric Association's Diagnostic and Statistical Manual. I was supposed to convert him to a heterosexual. My patient was about my age and very bright and he accepted my involvement because the department only charged him five dollars an hour. He told me in our opening interview that he had known about and accepted his homosexuality "as long as I can remember." He had some conflicts with authority that had cost him his latest job but said, "I'm fine with being a homosexual." So our goals for his therapy were in opposition from the start.

One night I saw him leaving the movie theater where we had both seen *Romeo and Juliet*. We nodded to each other. The next morning he began his hour by exclaiming his overwhelming desire for Romeo. I had had the same feelings toward Juliet. Later that day I talked to my supervisor Jim Delano who, in due course

8

became my analyst, and I told him that it was inappropriate for me to try to change my patient's sexuality. Instead, I would try to help him with his other conflicts. Open to being questioned Jim Delano agreed and, thankfully, so did the American Psychiatric Association a few years later.

Early Years at Rochester State Hospital

After Mayo I spent three years practicing at the state hospital in Rochester, Minnesota, beginning in 1962. The Rochester State Hospital was old and much had changed before I arrived there. I enjoyed reading the one hundred year-old records. I discovered that in the early days of psychiatry mental illnesses were thought to be caused by masturbation, so most of the men had a surgical procedure called "wiring." I could only imagine what that was. Paranoid delusions fit the times. For some early patients "Jesse James is after me" instead of the FBI would have run through their minds.

Some of the patients had been around forever. I started a state hospital newsletter and interviewed an old man who ran the chicken farm. "I've got five thousand birds," he said. He told me he had been committed in 1918 "because I had the D.T.'s." He could not remember ever seeing a doctor. "But I've got a good trailer, plenty to eat, and I like my work."

There were 5,500 patients in our hospital when I arrived. We had a dairy, a farm, greenhouses, and for many years, a limestone quarry. We still had a stonemason who worked with a crew of patients. Rochester was a rural community, and when severely mentally ill patients were admitted, they had a safe place to go and familiar work to do.

When I started work at the Rochester State Hospital, the superintendent Frank Tyce assigned me to the Women's Receiving Ward where all the female patients were admitted. I was also assigned to the Women's Receiving Ward West which contained most of the violent women, many of whom had "post-lobotomy syndrome." The Rochester State Hospital did hundreds of lobotomies during the 1940s, and many patients developed the syndrome

9

which is best described by all the Boy Scout virtues in reverse: "untrustworthy, unhelpful, unfriendly, etc." I was put in charge of managing these violent patients who were unquestionably damaged. The work I did was taxing but also fascinating.

On my first week I became acquainted with members of the staff. They told me that the women patients were separated from their families as they came into the building. Then they carried their bags into the unit where they were questioned, given a bath, and had a rectal temperature taken. I asked if any of them ever heard of somebody biting a thermometer. The men's receiving ward was attached to the women's. A male aide would come into the ward at meal times and shout, "Chow down!" I decided that all of this would change. The relatives would accompany the patients into our unit, see the rooms, and talk about their concerns with our staff. If there were no family, we would greet the patients and carry the bags into their rooms. No baths would be given and oral rather than rectal temperatures would be taken, and further, the male orderly was to come into the unit and address our female patients saying, "Ladies, dinner is served."

As my work there continued, I was perplexed when my charge nurse on morning rounds told me the night nurse had not given the nighttime medication I had prescribed, so I set my alarm clock for three in the morning and went to the unit and introduced myself to one startled night nurse and two aides. They had trouble believing that I was Dr. Rynearson. The night nurse said, "I've worked here for twenty-eight years, and I have never ever met a doctor." I went over my reasons for prescribing these drugs and told them if they had any questions, I would be glad to come back and answer them.

Another big change came next. On Receiving Ward West the nursing staff was locked in a room with a window so that terribly distressed patients could be observed, but the patients could see only what looked like nurses trapped in a closed cell. The feeling and look of the ward were captured very well in the movie *One Flew Over the Cuckoo's Nest.* I convinced Frank Tyce to redesign the unit so the nursing staff was placed in the center of the unit in an open station. The patients could then envision the nurses as caregivers rather than observers. I wanted to shift the emphasis from the patients somehow feeling like victims or being "kept" in an institution to a feeling of being cared for and nurtured.

Still, severe abuse of patients occurred in those days, and not just in "snake pits" as described in newspapers and movies. For example, I talked to one superintendent of the St. Peter State Hospital who told me that during pheasant season he invited his friends and family to hunt on the hospital farm using patients to drive the pheasants toward the hunters.

Back in the 1950s, before I arrived, they had only the promise of antipsychotic drugs that could return chronic mentally ill patients to the community. Frank Tyce had made it his goal to empty Rochester State Hospital. He believed that John F. Kennedy's new community mental health centers built in 1962 would provide better care. By 1965 our population was down from five thousand to under one thousand, and I urged Frank to take advantage of our relationship with the Mayo Clinic to provide state-of-the-art medical, neurological, and surgical service to Minnesota's mentally retarded patients, but he had determined to empty the hospital. Ten years later when the patient population dropped to 650, the state legislature saw no need for the hospital and turned it into a federal prison.

Moving to Scott & White

In 1965, eleven years after graduating from Harvard, I received a recruiting call from a doctor at Scott & White Clinic in Temple, Texas. At that time Scott & White had about forty doctors, a third of whom were Mayo-trained, and had just moved into a new building designed by a Mayo Clinic architect. Scott & White also modeled its internal organization after the Mayo Clinic, which was the first multi-specialty facility in the world where doctors of various specialties practiced together. They were salaried doctors working together for a patient's care, and each clinic conducted research and educational activities. Mayo has its own medical school; Scott & White is affiliated with Texas A&M University's medical school.

I was recruited to move to Texas because Dr. Sherve Frazier, chairman of the Department of Psychiatry at Baylor Medical School in Houston and Commissioner of Mental Health for the State of Texas, persuaded Scott & White's leaders that they needed a psychiatry department in order to be a "significant" multispecialty clinic. Dr. Frazier knew I had finished my residency program and suggested they contact me, and so I moved to Texas to begin a new psychiatry department.

Chapter Two
Insight Therapy and Repression

Prior to the late twentieth century, patients who were considered by their doctors or by the courts to be "a danger to themselves and others" were routinely committed to mental hospitals. Often these asylums for the insane were located in remote areas, further isolating psychiatric patients. "Out of mind, out of sight" could have been the motto for much of twentieth-century care. Despite the psychological knowledge mental health professionals gained from their education and their experience, my generation grew up in a culture that stigmatized mental illness.

Due to the stigma of psychiatric illness and the fear of developing it, psychiatric evaluations were confined to inpatient settings. Fifty years ago if patients were depressed, they were admitted to a psychiatric hospital or to the psychiatric unit of an academic medical center and spent the next two or three weeks undergoing a psychiatric evaluation during which social workers talked to the family, psychological testing was done, and a complete physical examination was conducted.

By the mid-twentieth century however, health care in general had embraced psychotherapy. Ideas articulated fifty years earlier by Freud, Jung, Adler, and others had percolated through the culture and had become honed and refined. Physicians and other mental health professionals had caught the wave of insight therapy and were ready to put these ideas to work to treat their patients. "Insight" is defined as "an understanding of the motivational forces behind one's actions, thoughts or behavior, self-knowledge." Therapy is "a curative power or quality." The insight, then, was believed to become the cure. Insight therapy would incorporate knowledge gained on the unconscious, "gut" level as opposed to intellectual, cognitive thinking. The influence of Sigmund Freud

13

cannot be overstated here.

Freud

Freud was a brilliant physician who was trained in medical school by, among others, a student of the great physiologist of the nineteenth century, Claude Bernard. Bernard is recognized as the most important mind in modern medicine and first associated illness with an imbalance within the cells. He proposed integration: the concept that a human has a constant internal environment maintained by a myriad-fold balancing and rebalancing, moving to relative stability called homeostasis. Freud recognized the importance of these dynamics and applied them to psychology. He believed internal forces were essential to provide mental equilibrium. He named these the id, the ego and the superego. For example, let's say you are walking down the street, and you see a beautiful diamond in a store window. You want it because it will make you more beautiful. Your id commands you to break the window, but your superego halts this action saying, "Thou shall not steal." Then your ego takes over and balances this conflict by working out a compromise: if you work hard and save enough money, you'll be able to buy it, perhaps on a layaway plan.

This conflict disrupts one's psychodynamics, or internal environment, and requires a constant balancing and rebalancing in order for a person to function successfully. For the well-educated and worldly upper-middle class at mid century, having a therapist or a psychoanalyst became a mark of status, and later the "human potential movement" promised that we could all lead more fulfilling lives and possibly spare the planet from war and environmental disaster if we only got rid of our hang-ups.

Although Freudian psychoanalysis was effective insight therapy, by the 1960s many psychiatrists were losing enthusiasm for his technique, partly because it required too much time and was too costly. Psychoanalysis was like Yap Island money: Yap Islanders used huge carved stone discs as money. Some stones were twelve feet in diameter and were leaned against boulders near the owners' homes. The value of this money was agreed upon, but it took so long to roll the "coin" to the place of barter that only a few could actually use it. Today, because of the success of new generations of psychopharmaceuticals in treating the symptoms of emotional illness and the sophistication of pharmaceutical companies in marketing these drugs to psychiatrists and directly to the public, insight therapy has nearly been eclipsed by use of medications. Like Yap money, insight therapy required too much energy and time.

Reviving Insight Therapy

Inpatient therapy has been virtually eliminated today. In the 1980s when the number of hospital beds for all specialties was being cut to the bone, psychiatric units were initially spared. However, by the 1990s almost all private psychiatric hospitals, including the celebrated Menninger, the Hartford Institute of Living, and Timberlawn in Dallas had either vanished or were vastly reduced in size. Insurance companies no longer covered long-term inpatient psychiatric care. The results have not always been for the best. For example, in 1996 I found myself in an emergency room at three in the morning with a psychotic, suicidal patient who was clearly a danger to himself and others. I had the phone to my ear arguing with a social worker in Baltimore about the insurance company for which she worked approving payment for the inpatient treatment the patient so obviously needed. Apparently a three-day waiting period was required for the patient to receive coverage.

As with other medical and surgical care, most psychiatric treatment in the early twenty-first century occurs in outpatient settings. This trend can be problematic in a number of ways including the underlying emphasis on cost containment rather than on doing what is best for each patient. But, with that said, some techniques of insight-oriented therapy adapt well to this new environment. Just as most mothers who experience a normal delivery don't need to spend three days recuperating on the maternity ward, most psychiatric patients don't need three months or even two weeks on the psychiatric unit. This big change in treatment does place added responsibility on the individual psychiatrist, however. The repressed emotions—emotions that have been delegated to the unconscious and underlie most illness, physical as well as mental—can be accessed in outpatient settings, but doing so, within today's compressed therapeutic schedules, requires techniques that go beyond conventional talk therapy.

Why do we need insight therapy at all? Despite the numerous criticisms of Freud's overall psychological theory, no one has discredited his then-revolutionary observation that emotional conflict is forcefully submerged from the conscious mind into the unconscious.

An adult brain constantly generates about twelve watts of electricity, enough to keep a flashlight glowing. If the inner conflict is severe and saps significant energy, the patient feels exhausted and drained of vitality. Perhaps one reason that young children have more energy than adults is that they have not learned to submerge emotional conflict. Adolescents, on the other hand, seem to struggle so hard with the normal pains associated with claiming their independence and strugglling with inner conflict that they may strike their parents and teachers as unaccountably exhausted.

My clinical experience has convinced me that at the moment of insight the patient has emotional release, feels a great weight lifted from his or her shoulders, and reports increased energy. My belief is that at this moment, energy is released from the repressive effort and made available for positive activities. Repression keeps the cause of the distress buried in the unconscious, but no matter how deeply it is submerged, this buried distress causes problems, and in my opinion, when those problems or physical symptoms appear, insight therapy is needed. A highway worker can use asphalt to cover a crack in a roadbed, but with the ordinary stress of traffic that weak spot will cause the highway to buckle, usually causing more damage than was there in the first place.

This does not mean that repression is an entirely negative phenomenon. Like many such things, it exists because it has an important function. In 1954 Will Durant pointed out in *The Story of*

Civilization that society can only survive if its members control their raw individual urges in exchange for the good of the group. Transmuting "violence into argument, murder into litigation," he noted, "has been part of the task of civilization."

The process of transmutation (becoming something different) requires that anti-social impulses be repressed (or as Durant pointed out, directed at other societies, as in war). Much of the time the repression is not all that selective. Feelings that might disrupt family stability or threaten a person's self-concept get buried as deeply as those that would threaten society–rampant lust, voracious greed, murderous rage. Being civilized requires repression.

Every one of us has a "dark side," a reservoir of repressed feelings. These, as I discovered at O'Connor's haberdashery, are represented literally by the appearance of our left facial profiles. Keeping this hidden self from view requires an enormous amount of energy. When we confront that self, that left side, we release that energy to the right side where it becomes available for creativity, intimacy, transcendent, spiritual, and aesthetic experiences and the feeling of well being.

In *Lost in the Cosmos* Walker Percy asks, "Why is it possible to learn more in ten minutes about the Crab Nebula Galaxy, which is 6,000 light years away, than you presently know about yourself, even though you've been stuck with yourself all your life?" Then Percy asks the reader to read the following statements carefully:

(a) You are extraordinarily generous, ecstatically loving of the right person, supremely knowledgeable about what is wrong with the country, about people, capable of moments of insight unsurpassed by any scientist or artist or writer in the country. You possess an infinite potentiality.

(b) You are of all people in the world probably the most selfish, hateful, envious (e.g., you take pleasure in reading death notices in the newspaper and hearing of an acquaintance's heart attack), the most treacherous, the most frightened and above all the phoniest.

(c) You are neither of the above.

(d) You are both of the above.

17

"Now," Percy continues, "answer this question as honestly as you can. Which of these more nearly describes you?" Sixty percent of the respondents checked "Both," and Percy's answer to this is "We are both." Only by recognizing this essential truth of the human condition and embracing our hidden selves can we heal the pain of being divided. It is this pain that saps the brain's energy and produces symptoms that often send us to the physician.

Each of us has within us a common enemy. It may have different faces, but it always has a similar identity—a sense of alienation, being incomplete, inauthentic, and divorced from ourselves. We expend so much energy on keeping our "dark side" locked away that we have little left over for love, joy, learning, and creativity. But this doesn't have to be a mandatory life sentence. By recognizing and accepting our feeling side, and then by truly experiencing it, we can release more energy to fuel joy and transcendence. This is not to say that other kinds of treatment, including the use of psychoactive medications, aren't important. In many mental illnesses such as schizophrenia, manic-depressive disorder, obsessive-compulsive disorder, depression, and anxiety disorders, medications are often extremely effective when prescribed and managed by psychiatrists.

Regressive Shock

During my junior year in medical school, I had my first rotation on a psychiatric unit. It was a terrible experience. A research psychiatrist on a Central Intelligence Agency grant was experimenting with a dozen patients to test the effects of Ewing Cameron's technique called regressive shock. Our group was to follow these patients to see if ten to twelve shock treatments a day would cause a regression to an infantile stage in which the patient could not eat, speak, or move in a coordinated way. They had to regress to the point where they had what's called a positive Babinski sign, a sign present in an infant whereby if the sole of the baby's foot is scratched, the big toe goes up. Once regressed to this stage, a team of nurses was to repeatedly tell them positive things: "You're a good person, people love you." This was supposed to replace any past negative input with positive thoughts.

On reading Naomi Klein's book *The Shock Doctrine* a few months ago, I was reminded of my introduction to psychiatry. She described a tri-national meeting in 1951 of intelligence agencies and academics to discuss how Communists had discovered brainwashing. They were interested in how Russians had caused American soldiers captured in Korea to issue complete confessions without physical torture. Present were Dr. Ewing Cameron, head of the Department of Psychiatry at McGill, and the head psychologist, Donald Hebb, Director of Psychology at McGill. Dr. Hebb speculated that sensory deprivation would be an effective "de-patterning" process. He had paid McGill students to be isolated from all sensory input, including encasing their limbs and hands so they could not feel. All of the students became psychotic in hours or days, and four of them described this as torture. Hebb then declared this was a clear violation of medical ethics.

Dr. Cameron proceeded enthusiastically because he wanted a violent destruction of the brain to totally de-pattern patients in order to create the Aristotelian *tabula rasa* (clean slate) where there are no memories. Naomi Klein reports that the CIA, which was funding Dr. Cameron's research, was later successfully sued by some of the subjects of the project.

The initial part of my first psychotherapy rotation dealt with the research on regressive shock, and the second half was on beginning psychotherapy taught by Dr. Raymond Parker. When I discussed the regressive shock research with Dr. Parker, he was appalled that we had been exposed to that and said he would try to block the research program through the chairman of our medical school's psychiatry department. Shortly after this meeting Dr. Parker resigned. The CIA's grant must have trumped compassionate care, and now this technique is one of the mainstays of America's torture program. This was my introduction to psychiatry.

However, there can be a positive place for electroshock treatments (EST). The idea of EST repels many people. It seems to be an unscientific, barbaric treatment, an assault on the brain. At one time I, too, couldn't believe EST could be beneficial, but I know

19

now it is by far the safest and most effective treatment for patients who have not responded to all other treatments and suffer severe depression and mania. I have told my wife, my personal physician, and my colleagues that if I suffer from either of these, I want them to give me EST.

Severe depression is so dreadful that the sufferer has no words to describe it. The author William Styron comes close in his book *Darkness Visible*, a description of the writer's descent into madness and depression, from which he later recovered. The title is taken from John Milton's reference of Hell in *Paradise Lost*. In my first month of training in St. Mary's Hospital at the Mayo Clinic, I was assigned a patient named Mrs. Larson, a sixty-eight year-old wife of a retired minister from Mason City, Iowa. The day after her husband retired, they left Iowa to drive to a northern Minnesota resort for their first real vacation. Shortly after leaving Mason City she became mute and unresponsive, which frightened her husband, so he stopped at St. Mary's emergency room. Since the doctor could not communicate with her, he began a physical examination. He looked in her mouth and saw hemorrhages on her tonsils. He then undid the scarf around her neck and was alarmed by the deep rope burns he had exposed. She was then admitted to the psychiatry unit and assigned to me.

As I introduced myself, I looked into her eyes and saw the depth of her despair. Because she was such a severe suicide risk, we completed her medical examination and then we began electroshock treatments. After the fifth treatment, she began applying her makeup. After the eighth treatment, she said she was well and eager to continue her trip north. She had no idea why she attempted suicide but said, "I thank God for breaking the rope."

Every two years the Texas Legislature meets, and at each session there is present, always, an anti-EST group that demands a law banning these treatments. The Texas Psychiatric Association makes certain our views are represented. On one such occasion a petitioner stated that Ernest Hemingway's brain was destroyed by EST at the Mayo Clinic. I told him I was in the psychiatric unit at the time of Hemingway's treatment and dismissal. Hemingway had received a series of electroshock treatments, and afterward

20

he was mentally clear and in good spirits. In fact, we had become friends (he used to call me his sparring partner) during his stay in Rochester, and he came to our house for dinner the night before he left. During dinner he invited us to join him on his next fishing trip. We also talked about his terror of another severe depression. This had been his second admission to the psychiatric unit, and both visits had been before the availability of mood stabilizers such as lithium. He remembered how he felt when he had checked into the hospital and said he never wanted to feel that way again.

Chapter Three
Resistance to Psychiatry

I became a psychiatrist because I find people fascinating. The more I understood, the more I wanted to know. Treating a person for emotional distress is like being a geologist who drills a core sample through strata laid down over the years, one on top of the other, each different, each revealing something new, each deepening the understanding of how the layers above helped create the present hills and valleys.

By the time I completed my junior year in medical school, I had made up my mind that I would finish my degree and then paddle my canoe up a different river. But two extraordinary experiences at Mayo that summer between my third and fourth years of medical school changed the course of my professional life. Both experiences came from repressed inner conflict.

The first occurred with Dr. Dick Steinhilber, known as Steinie, who was famous for treating the students and residents to coffee and doughnuts after rounds. One morning he told the team about his own experience with repressed conflict. He told us about a terrible fight he had with his wife Louise. Without her knowledge, Steinie had bought what we called the Woltman house, one of the grandest on "Pill Hill," Rochester's rich doctor neighborhood. He had expected Louise to be pleased, but instead she was furious. Here was a decision that would affect every aspect of her daily life, and he had not consulted her. It was as if her feelings were irrelevant. At one point she had even mentioned divorce.

Steinie told us that at a critical moment he had an important insight. He realized that his father had never been able to provide his mother with the large house she had always wanted. It then occurred to him that he was buying the Woltman house for his mother and not his wife and that is why he hadn't involved Louise in the decision and also why it had been so important to him. When he shared this insight with her, she understood and forgave him. They moved into the Woltman house and resumed a comfortable relationship.

Later that morning, I had the second life-changing experience. I went to the orthopedic ward to see a young man with intractable back pain. His pain was so severe that he was rigid in bed. Unable to find anything physically wrong that could cause such agony, the orthopedist had requested a psychiatry consultation. When I entered the room, the young man asked what service I represented. I told him psychiatry, and to my surprise he asked if I had any tissues. Returning with a box, I sat down next to him. He grabbed a fistful and began to sob. After ten minutes, he sat up, took another wad of tissues and sobbed for another ten minutes. Then he looked at me and said, "I've got a terrible conflict. I'm supposed to get married in three weeks, and there's something I haven't told my fiancée, my family, or even myself. I'm homosexual. I know I should tell her, but I haven't been able to. I was planning to kill myself, but the pain immobilized me, so I couldn't do it."

After a long pause the young man added, "I think I can tell her now. Thank you so much." He stood up smoothly, apparently free of pain, and began assembling his belongings. I hadn't said a word. When I left the room, the orthopedist asked me what had happened. I said, "Your patient is well. He's free of pain."

The orthopedist asked, "How did you do that?"

I replied, "I don't know."

When I reported my consultation to Steinie the next morning he declared, "Now you know the answer. Don't just say something, sit there!" In psychotherapy "sitting there" translates into listening—fully attentive, nonjudgmental listening. Although I may have gone without uttering a word, I had to be completely focused on the young man with the back pain, not planning a slide presentation for Tuesday's staff meeting or wondering whether the sluggish start that morning meant the car needed a tune-up, and not thinking about the next appointment. My listening enabled him to discover, and express his repressed feelings. I soon discovered that as soon as my attention shifted, patients could tell, and the therapeutic momentum stalled; but once patients sensed that I was fully present, listening attentively, most would slide naturally onto the narrative path. We all need empathic attention to be fully affirmed and understood.

24

Another memorable part of my six weeks as a Mayo extern was attending rounds with Dr. Robert Faucet, a psychiatrist who specialized in hospital consultations. He worked with Mayo general internists and specialists, so he had the advantage of being recognized as a "real doctor."

Faucet had begun his career as a board-certified internist and had switched to psychiatry because he became fascinated with the underlying conflicts that led to so many chronic, hard-to-treat conditions. Being a consulting psychiatrist at Mayo allowed him to help patients and his physician colleagues ferret out the origins of persistent gastroenteritis and intractable back pain.

On rounds one morning we trooped onto the gastrointestinal service where Bob interviewed a meek, forty-something accountant who was having difficulty swallowing. There was no medical explanation for the man's symptom. Bob asked the patient to tell him a bit about himself. Once the man had said where he lived and worked, he began talking about his personal relationships. His mother had complained constantly, and his father had been emotionally absent. Dinnertime had been tense. He and his sister couldn't leave the table until they had "joined the Clean Plate Club."

When he was seventeen, his mother died from complications of multiple sclerosis. His troubles continued into adulthood. As Bob's patient spoke, he revealed himself as an obsessive and passive individual, tyrannized by a mean-spirited boss and a demanding disabled wife. His trouble swallowing had begun when his adored seventeen-year-old daughter, the one light in his life, became pregnant by the choir director at his church. He took the situation to the church's minister who had been the main source of emotional support helping the patient cope with his miserable existence at work and at home, but the minister refused to discipline the choir director.

As the patient spoke he began sobbing, and all of us on the team were moved to tears listening to his story. The cause of the symptom was clear as was the prescription. The patient needed to get off the GI (gastroenterology) service and get into psychotherapy. The whole process had taken less than forty-five minutes.

25

Later, when Bob Faucet met with the gastroenterologist, he told the man's tragic story and outlined the underlying psychodynamics ending with: "He just couldn't swallow any more."

The gastroenterologist replied, "Then I'll tell him to eat his big meal at noon rather than at night." He obviously did not get it. Unable to believe what I had heard, as soon as we were off the GI floor, I asked Bob how he could stand doing consultations like that day after day when he got "big meal at noon" comments. He smiled wanly and told me, "It's like driving pilings into deep mud. Once in awhile you'll hit something solid." On that day with Bob Faucet I knew that psychiatry was my field. I also knew I wanted to practice in a multi-specialty clinic, so when Scott & White invited me to start a psychiatry department, I headed south. Although I knew it might be difficult to find Bob Faucet's "something solid," I did not expect as much resistance from the doctors within the institution as I found.

Resistance to Psychiatry from Doctors

Resistance lingered, both among the Mayo staff and among patients and their families. I should have recalled a cautionary conversation I had with Dr. Frank Braceland, past president of the American Psychiatric Association. In 1946 the Mayo Clinic had recruited him as their first psychiatrist. When they established the multi-specialty clinic in 1889, William and Charles Mayo specified that there were two kinds of patients they didn't want to treat: those with tuberculosis and those with psychiatric disorders. Either, they reasoned, would scare off other patients. It took almost six decades for the policy toward the latter to change.

Braceland said that when he first arrived at Mayo, one of his colleagues called and asked him to see the physician's wife. Frank said, "I'll be glad to. Bring her in."

"I'd rather you didn't see her at the clinic," his fellow practitioner said. "Could you come to the house?"

"Certainly," Braceland replied.

"Could you come in the evening?" The physician specified a time after dusk. Braceland agreed. "I hope," said the doctor, "you

26

won't mind if I don't leave the porch light on."

Later, when I joined the Scott & White staff as the first psychiatrist, the resistance to psychiatry was not that extreme, but neither was it completely free of the bias and stigma that even doctors attached to psychiatric disorders and to those of us who specialized in them.

With my usual enthusiasm I arrived in Texas certain of self and mission. Unaware of the resistance from my fellow physicians, I could not understand why so many of my suggestions were shelved, so much of what I needed in order to build the department shunted aside. "We don't do things that way at Scott & White" became the usual response to my requests. Much of the push-back came from two members of the clinic's seven-member board of directors. I later learned that they had tried to keep the president, Olin Gober, from hiring me. One was Dr. Robert A. Murray, chairman of the Department of Orthopedics. The other was the head of surgery. To them, psychiatry was not real medicine, and psychiatrists were not real doctors.

Conversion Symptoms

A few weeks after I arrived, Dr. Murray sent me a patient named Mr. Walker. He was a pale man in his early fifties, and his most notable characteristic was his posture. He was severely hunched, doubled over as if he bore the weight of the world on his shoulders. I marveled that he could even walk. Despite all of Bob Murray's orthopedic knowledge and skill, his attempts to treat the man had failed. From the way he had described the case, I could tell that Bob expected me to fail, too.

When Mr. Walker and his wife entered my office, I knew that he had a rare condition called camptocormia, a type of hysterical conversion from emotional repression to physical symptoms that is always symbolic of a deeper issue. While this is a genuine neurological problem, it most frequently shows up as an hysterical conversion disorder, the patient manifesting emotional pain as physical pain. I had seen only one other case during my neurology rotation at Mayo, but the symptoms of this disorder are so distinc-

27

tive that I was certain of my diagnosis. His wife was a frightened little woman, frantic, and always on the phone asking Dr. Murray to do more. She was a very religious woman and constantly read articles about cures, sometimes insisting that Mr. Walker see other healers. When I asked about the first sign of symptoms, Mrs. Walker said she thought it had started about fifteen years before with some illness, but she was not sure. Mr. Walker thought it was an infection, and he had crumpled over and just stayed that way. Neither could remember what might have happened, but they both told me they were desperate for a cure.

As I took his history, I was convinced that his symptom had outlived its protective usefulness. I asked if his condition kept him from doing anything, but he said it didn't. I said, "If there was no reason for you to stay the way you are, I think I can cure your symptom. If we can agree that this is caused by some emotional block, and if you believe you can be cured by hypnosis, then it will work."

All patients diagnosed as hysterics are highly suggestible people, and only a suggestible individual can manufacture a symbolic symptom. Being suggestible makes hysterics excellent subjects for hypnosis because hypnosis works by having the subject accept a suggestion. Mr. Walker was no exception. He went into the hypnotic trance in about three minutes. While he was under, I suggested that his emotional block had disappeared and that he could walk normally. On the count of three, he awoke, jumped up from his chair, and began prancing around the room. Breaking into tears Mrs. Walker fell on her knees, thanking Jesus. As the Walkers left, I asked them to do me a favor. "Oh, anything, Dr. Rynearson," they replied in unison.

"Please stop by Dr. Murray's office and thank him for the referral." They did. And from that day forward Bob Murray's resistance disappeared, and he gave his whole-hearted support to the clinic's new psychiatry department.

About this same time, the head of surgery referred a man to me who had been admitted for severe epigastric pain (acid-induced gastric distress). Although the pain involved the area just above the stomach, the site of most peptic ulcers, it was uncharacteristic of that disorder because it radiated from his upper abdomen back to the area between his shoulder blades.

The surgeon had decided that the patient's problem was depression and expected me to concur with his diagnosis. But after interviewing the man and conducting psychological tests, I was convinced that he was not depressed. At Mayo I had studied referred pain—pain that is experienced in one place when the cause is in another. For example, a patient having a heart attack may feel pain in his jaw. This patient fit the picture of a referred-pain pattern caused by a peptic ulcer on the posterior wall of the duodenum. When I told the surgeon I thought his patient suffered not from depression, but from an ulcer a foot away from where he felt the pain, the surgeon was incredulous. "You mean you think I should operate on this man?" he asked.

"You are the surgeon," I said, "but in my opinion, you should operate." He did operate, and I was relieved when the surgery confirmed my diagnosis, and although the surgeon never stopped testing me, he stopped opposing me at every turn. By demonstrating the potential of psychiatry to cure patients' chronic symptoms and to screen out mental illness when the cause of a symptom truly was physical, I had hit two home runs in the bottom of the first inning. Now I could start the real work of building the department.

Generally, no one came to Scott & White complaining of psychiatric problems. My practice involved seeing patients referred to me by colleagues in other specialties who suspected (usually correctly) that a physical complaint might have an emotional component. A cardiologist unable to find a defect to explain a racing heart would ask me to evaluate the patient for anxiety disorder. An orthopedist would call me in on a case of mysterious back pain. Although those referrals remained a major part of our department's practice, we gradually began to see patients who came to Scott & White for depression, eating disorders, and other psychiatric complaints.

As chair of the department, I supervised care for hundreds of patients a year. In addition to my administrative duties, my typical day involved initial evaluations with new patients, individual and group sessions with psychiatric outpatients, rounds on inpatients, and consultations in the emergency room and with medical and surgical patients who were having trouble coping emotionally with serious illnesses or injuries.

An indication of my colleagues' acceptance of psychiatry came soon enough. Late one night shortly after I had arrived at Scott & White, I was called in to manage an emergency in the hospital. When I arrived, a middle-aged, balding, red-headed man was screaming into a phone while a voluptuous blonde woman was loudly demanding that nurses bring him more whiskey. The patient was a internationally known celebrity, His attending physician had been treating his delirium tremens (DT's) with whiskey. (Before we had detox drugs like Librium and Valium, one of the treatments for DT's was alcohol in decreasing doses.) I dismissed everyone but the man from the room, took away his phone, and started him on a Librium detox. It turned out that the woman who had been supplying him with alcohol had stopped giving it to him four days before he came into the hospital, so he was in severe withdrawal. When he recovered from his delirium tremens, he left before anyone could give him a complete medical workup.

That I was trusted to handle this potentially high-profile case told me that acceptance within the medical community was coming.

Most patients arrived with their own resistance to psychotherapy. This is easy to spot. A well-educated patient may challenge the method or approach engaging in what I call "playing chess." Or a patient may say that he or she "just can't remember; it was so long ago." Another way resistance expresses itself is in externalizing the inner conflict, that is, blaming other people or situations in the outer world. Such projection makes the patient feel less responsible for his or her problems but conversely, less able to do anything about them. It was important for me to find a way to reduce that resistance, and I found art to be a remarkably effective tool.

Within a year of my arrival, I added a creative art program that was highly effective in helping patients overcome resistance to insight. Because the patient created the drawing, painting, or poem,

30

he or she could not escape ownership of its content. For example, if a woman told me that she did not mean to draw her mother as taller than her father and argued that he really was a lot bigger, I could reply, "But you did." Most of my therapeutic relationships followed a similar pattern. During the first few sessions using art and other techniques, the patient and I could break through some resistance. The middle sessions were devoted to seeing the patterns in the family and accepting that what the patient had experienced had been present in the family, repeated over and over again, with each new generation assuming the same old roles. For patients to recognize this was usually highly motivating. Not only did patients want to escape this cycle, but also they wanted to be sure their children did not follow it. We devoted the last sessions to applying these insights to the patient's present life and future life and to celebrating the patient's relief at having the weight of the repressed memories lifted from his or her shoulders.

Learning from My Patients

In addition, each patient also taught me a little bit about myself. Consider the case of Betsy James. All of us experience pain, sorrow, rejection, and disappointments in our lives. For some of us emotional distress is more exaggerated. Betsy was twenty-four and the daughter of a prominent Dallas family. She had been seen by an internist for agitation and fine tremors, common symptoms of an overactive thyroid, and she was having hallucinations. She heard threatening voices and saw evil people attacking her. Betsy's life was a waking nightmare. The internist referred her to me, and I admitted her to the psychiatric unit. Betsy admitted that she regularly took recreational drugs, among them marijuana, heroin, and LSD. My initial assessment resulted in a complicated diagnosis: schizophrenia and hyperthyroidism exacerbated by substance addiction. At least she had the presence of mind to steer clear of amphetamines. Given her thyroid condition, speed could have killed her.

Betsy wrote extraordinary lyrical free verse filled with vivid images. I stopped by her room several times a day either for scheduled individual therapy sessions or as impromptu visits after rounds. I did so to check on her progress, but also to enjoy her latest poem. On one particular morning after she had been on the unit for about a week, I figured I could shoehorn in a visit with her before my first outpatient clinic appointment. But there was no new poem that day. I found Betsy extremely agitated, responding to threatening auditory and visual hallucinations. Although she had seemed to be improving the day before, on this day she was terrified. I spent forty-five minutes reassuring her until she began to calm down. Then I remembered my first outpatient, whom I imagined was cooling her heels in my waiting room. I pulled my great-grandfather's pocket watch from the right pocket of my white doctor's coat, opened up the case, and looked at the time. Betsy looked at me and said, "I'm late! I'm late, for a very important date!" quoting *Alice in Wonderland's* White Rabbit.

I must have borne an uncanny resemblance to the illustration in the familiar edition of that children's classic: white coat, glasses, and huge pocket watch. There I was, preparing to race off to my next appointment when what I should have been doing was staying with her as long as she needed me. And she knew that, too. The next morning, I stashed the pocket watch where it belonged, among my family mementos. I was still learning how important it was just to take time to listen.

Chapter Four
Repressed Emotional Conflict and the Symptoms

Earlier Twentieth Century Treatment

In my practice, I discovered the patient's chief complaint was seldom the actual problem. Whether the chronic complaint was fatigue, back pain, irritable bowel syndrome, difficulty sleeping, or severe headache, it was likely to be only a secondary symptom of an underlying problem. In case after case the root cause was a repressed emotional conflict.

When Dad joined the Mayo Clinic in 1927, the practice of medicine was very different than today; there were very few medical specialists, and there was quite limited technology. Most physicians were general practitioners who had spent their lives in small communities trying to understand their patients. They knew each family's secrets and could effectively sort out those few patients whose life stresses did not explain their symptoms. They treated the simple fractures and fevers. The complicated cases they referred to specialists. My father, a fellow in endocrinology, admired these generalists greatly, even more so after a house call he made one stormy winter night. He was taking his turn covering the phone when it rang.

"Are you the doctor on call?" a woman asked.

My father said, "Yes."

"Pa's a-fittin'," the caller said. "Ya have to come out." She gave him directions to her farm twelve miles outside Rochester on the Minnesota prairie. "I'll leave a kerosene lamp on the mailbox and put the dogs up."

"There's a blizzard outside," my father said. "I don't think I ought to go."

"Oughta?" the woman shouted. "Ya gotta!"

Braving the storm, Dad drove the clinic's Model A Ford to the farmer's house. When he entered he saw a husky man clutching the leg of the iron wood burning stove, which he, in his tonic-clonic pseudo-seizure, had wrenched from the wall. He was a fittin', all right. Ashes and smoke were everywhere, and the dogs were howling in the bedroom where the family had taken refuge. My father injected the farmer in each buttock, right through his overalls with four cubic centimeters (cc's) of paraldehyde, the powerful and at that time only available sedative. In a few minutes the farmer relaxed and began to sob. My dad asked him what had happened. "I lost all our money to the slots," the farmer confessed. Slowly the family ventured out of the bedroom. The farmer told his wife about his gambling loss, and she forgave him.

Rather than venture out again into the storm, my dad stayed until dawn. By the time the sun rose, peace had returned to the farmhouse. The farmer's chief complaint–his fit–was the symptom, not the real problem. Sizing up the situation quickly, my father had recognized the need to look for the cause in some repressed emotional conflict, and additionally, he gave the patient an invaluable healing tool—time.

For years my father told and retold the tale of the storm, the farmer who was a-fittin' and the profound way the incident affected my father's sense of self. "On that night," my father liked to conclude his story, "I really felt like a 'real doctor.' " In my childhood the story took on the power of a profound family myth, a truth that demanded to be pondered. A basic truth in the story, one not entirely lost on me, was that for me, becoming a real doctor involved finding the right time to listen in order to discover the patient's repressed conflicts causing his or her symptoms.

The patients whom doctors saw in the early twentieth century were just like those treated by their counterparts today although the actual repressed experiences that often prompted these symptoms have varied from era to era and culture to culture. Regardless of the specific content of the emotional conflict, or of the specific behaviors that threatened patients' sense of themselves, the mechanism of repression has remained the same across centuries and continents.

Because the early twentieth-century doctors almost always knew the patient personally, sometimes had delivered them, and frequently treated the same people for a decade or more, they

34

could tell when a patient walked into the office whether there had been a change. Did he or she look sick or angry? The physicians and patients were part of the same small neighborhood, so the doctors were aware of most of the stresses the patients were under. If the woman who owned the corner store had lost her mother two months before, the doctor knew it. In fact, the doctor would probably have treated the mother and attended her funeral. In those days physicians had plenty of office time to devote to discussing their patients' problems.

These doctors also understood how to employ the power attached to medical ritual. Malcomb Rody, my wife's uncle, was a general practitioner in a little prairie town in Iowa. He had on hand in his office all the basic ingredients of most early twentieth-century medicines. Rather than handing a patient a prescription to be filled at the nearest pharmacy, he would mix the compound right there in his office, often using his well-worn mortar and pestle to crush herbs and minerals into a powder with the patient looking on. Witnessing this ritual heightened the always powerful placebo effect, which is a well-documented adjunct to the effectiveness of any drug. To boost it even further, Uncle Rody would give his patient detailed instructions for the medication's use. For example, each dose of a powder for headaches would be wrapped in a carefully folded piece of paper. The patient would be instructed to dissolve the contents in warm water with a teaspoon of vinegar and drink it half an hour before meals and again at bedtime.

Uncle Rody had a special salve for Bell's palsy, the usually painless but disfiguring ailment of the nerve controlling the muscles on one side of the face. Grinding up the chemicals with his mortar and pestle and stirring them into an oily base, he sent the patient home with the compound and instructions to rub the salve into the face clockwise, twice daily, one hundred times. "Do this morning and night for a month," he said.

After a couple of weeks, the patient would call him in distress to say, "I can't remember whether I rubbed the salve clockwise or counterclockwise this morning. What should I do?" Uncle Rody would reply, "I'm afraid you'll just have to start over. Count this as Day One, and apply the compound for another month. And it's clockwise."

Left alone, the facial nerve regenerates at the rate of about an inch a month. In whatever direction it is applied, massage may help. It certainly does not hurt. I have never read of a particular chemical formula that affects the recovery rate, but I have witnessed many cases of the placebo effect speeding healing. Canadian physician William Osler, one of the four founders of Johns Hopkins Medical School and the author of *The Principles and Practice of Medicine*, the dominant medical textbook worldwide for more than fifty years, understood this fully.

One day in the late 1800s, Osler was summoned immediately after a lecture to the home of a sick child. Still wearing his full academic robes, garb today's professors of medicine reserve for formal occasions such as commencements, he arrived to find the little boy weak and burning with fever. The child had stopped eating, and his father was losing hope. Without antibiotics or even aspirin to treat the child, Osler asked the boy's father to bring him a peach and some sugar. Pulling out his pocketknife, Dr. Osler carefully sliced the peach. Dipping each slice in sugar, he told the little boy that it was a magic fruit that would make him well. As he coaxed him to eat, the boy's eyes became focused and lost some of their cloudy quality. He seemed quite taken by Dr. Osler's professorial regalia.

Dr. Osler left, telling the boy and his father that he would be back the next day. He returned at the same time every day for a week clad in his robes and repeated the ritual with the peach. To the father's surprise and joy the little boy recovered. The chief ingredients in his treatment had been Osler's compassionate attention and the conviction he projected that the child could get well. Earlier medicine and health relied on empathy and compassion and understanding the patient in order to unlock repressed emotions causing illness or slowing healing. Doctors often understood and relied upon the connection between the patients' emotions and their physical symptoms for healing.

Since William Osler's time medical technology and pharmacology have changed dramatically, but human beings are much the same as they were then. Although our medical ancestors placed

36

more emphasis on loosening constipated bowels than practitioners do today, blocked emotions still play a key role in most complaints, physical as well as psychological.

In 1900 Western medicine possessed few drugs and little technical equipment. Doctors had morphine to treat pain, cascara to alleviate constipation, scalpels and clamps for appendicitis. But the use of these was limited. Before antibiotics, surgery was highly hazardous due to the risk of infection. The great physicians of the day were renowned for practicing the art of medicine, using their intuition and communication skills to heal their frightened patients. These doctors took the time to listen and understand the physical problem and to remedy the inner conflict that often underlay it.

The March 2006 issue of the newsletter "Scott and White Today" contained an article by our staff librarian, June Lubowinski, about the early days of our pharmacy. She listed the main drugs in use in 1900:

> Morphine, strychnine, whiskey, opium, carbolic acid, bichloride of mercury and cascara. This is a small group of therapeutic substances when you realize that two of these preparations were used primarily for cleaning and sterilizing equipment. In a time when making the patient comfortable was as important as any medicine they had to give, warmth, nourishment and clean surroundings were the gold standard of therapy. In addition, we are told that mineral oil was liberally administered, and more often patients were given a large dose of compassionate listening, which is still the best medicine available.

Psychological or Physical Illness?

Twenty-first-century physicians, in contrast, have at hand a superabundance of space-age technologies and thousands of powerful pharmaceuticals. When one of my dearest friends was in his eighties, he developed congestive heart failure along with the early stages of senile dementia. His cardiologist suggested surgery to replace his mitral and aortic valves. Given the risks of

37

major heart surgery for a man his age, his wife argued against it. His children, however, wanted to "do something for Dad," so my friend signed the consent form.

Although the surgery did improve his heart function, my friend never recovered consciousness. He slid into a persistent vegetative state. His children could not bear to visit him, but during the weeks he took to die his wife sat at his bedside. Every shift his cardiologist or a resident would come in, greet her politely, look at the monitors tracking his vital signs, and leave saying, "Things are looking good" or "Everything looks fine." Finally, one morning she stood up and demanded, "For God's sake, look at the patient. Don't just look at the machines!"

Experienced clinicians know that eighty to ninety percent of patients today given advanced tests such as CT scans, X-rays, MRIs, and so on, do not need them. They need time from their doctor and need to be listened to. Of course, some patients in recent years insist on having all the tests in the biomedical arsenal "just in case." For one thing, there is no financial incentive to do otherwise. Those with insurance are not paying for the scans and biopsies directly because the procedures were covered. For another, patients may unconsciously prefer that something "real" and serious be identified as the cause of their distress, rather than having to confront a long-buried emotional issue. In 1934, pioneer American psychiatrist, Karl Menninger, in his paper "Polysurgery and Polysurgerical Addiction" published in *Psychoanalytic Quarterly*, observed that patients would rather hear that they have a condition requiring a daunting surgery than one that threatens their psychological defenses. Unless the individual was brittle with marginal psychological defenses, a situation that often arose with psychotics, he or she would unconsciously seek the dependent role of the sick person. This was, in fact, the main reason why so many patients resisted their physicians' attempts to cure them.

Patients who were threatened by loss of control were frightened that they might lose their emotional integrity. If all of their emotional defenses were stripped away, or failed them, they felt overwhelming anxiety. But when this happened, they seldom

38

shattered into little pieces. Instead, they regressed into a dependent position, becoming sick, so that they could receive nurturing. I saw that happen with my own father.

For Dad, an endocrinologist, the single affirmation of his value was becoming a member of the Mayo Clinic Board of Governors. When he was fifty-five it looked like he had a sure shot at this coveted position. Every few years two members would cycle off the board, and the board would recommend two staff physicians to replace them. In the past the clinic staff had always ratified the board's choice, but the staff had begun to chafe at being thought of as nothing more than a rubber stamp. Sensing this, the board took pains to nominate two doctors who were extremely popular with the staff—my father and a well-liked general surgeon.

Unfortunately, a sizable contingent among the staff was not so much concerned about the characteristics of the individuals brought forth as they were about the closed process. Rebelling, they nominated two doctors from the floor and elected them. Stunned that he had lost, my father experienced an acute flare-up of his chronic shoulder pain. The ache had not stopped him from hunting and fishing, but after the lost election, it suddenly became disabling. He told a surgeon colleague that he needed an operation without delay, and the surgeon agreed. Dad took a long time recovering from the surgery, and during those many weeks, the institution that had rejected him had to nurture him. Fortunately, the surgery did my father no harm. In fact, it provided an excuse for a much-needed rest and an opportunity to put his career into perspective. He responded to the treatment, and he escaped complications.

Occasionally, however, a patient with an emotional problem may actually have a serious physical condition as well. When the symptoms are similar, one can mask the other, resulting in an outcome that is deeply distressing for both patient and therapist. I'd been at Scott & White only a couple of years when a neurologist colleague referred such a patient to me. My colleague attached one of his typically brusque and unequivocal notes to her chart: "Patient has negative neurological exam. Her complaint of weakness in her left hand represents a conversion reaction. She has unconsciously converted her real problem into a 'weak hand.' Please evaluate and treat. No need for her to return to neurology."

As the consulting psychiatrist, I was expecting a defensive, resistant patient, but Mrs. Chetowski was anything but that. "I'm relieved," she told me. "I was sure I had a brain tumor." In my psychiatric evaluation, I searched for an internalized conflict that could have caused the weakness. Conversion symptoms always have an important symbolic meaning. A patient who was conflicted by something he or she saw, heard or might say, could become blind, deaf, or dumb—an unconscious version of the famous three Chinese monkeys.

My search proved fruitful, or so I thought. Mrs. Chetowski told me that her hand weakness had begun three months earlier on the day she remembered it was the anniversary of her father's death. When I asked for details of his death, she sobbed as she told the story of his suicide. She was a senior in high school, and he had just dropped her off at a friend's house. She walked around to the driver's side to kiss him goodbye. He rolled down the window and kissed her, transferred a pistol from his right hand to his left, and shot himself in the head. "He used his left hand because he didn't want to hurt me," she explained. "Aha!" I thought, "the left hand."

As our interview concluded, she told me the tears had helped "and my left hand is stronger." We scheduled regular appointments and after several weeks, Mrs. Chetowski's husband, the mayor of a nearby town, phoned to tell me of her continuing improvement. He said that both he and his eight-year-old son were grateful.

Mrs. Chetowski's therapy revealed significant emotional trauma. Her father had abused her sexually from the time she was eight until her junior year in high school when she finally told her mother. Her confession set in motion an angry confrontation between her parents, her father's expression of remorse, and less than a year later, his suicide. "If I had just kept everything to myself," she said with sorrow.

But despite her progress in psychotherapy, her symptoms did not improve. Mrs. Chetowski's left hand may have felt stronger to her, but I could not tell the difference when I asked her to squeeze my hand. In addition, she was experiencing severe headaches and, on two occasions, double vision. I sent her back to my neurologist colleague who repeated the electroencephalogram (EEG) skull films and his clinical neurological exams. He found her "neurologically intact." Before the CAT scans, PET scans, and MRIs that now allow us to literally see inside the brain and watch it function, we depended on the neurologist's clinical experience to differentiate diseases of the central nervous system from psychiatric disorders.

Early one morning Mr. Chetowski called me at home to report that his wife had suffered a seizure in her sleep. She had bitten her tongue and had lost control of her bladder and bowels. He brought her to the emergency room where I assessed her. Although she was slightly confused, she appeared well and insisted that she was fine. Clearly she was not. Conversion disorders can take many forms, but a grand mal seizure during sleep is not one of them. I told the Chetowskis that I wanted another neurologist's opinion. I arranged to have a well-regarded specialist in Dallas see her, and he discovered a deeply seated and inoperable brain tumor. Mrs. Chetowski's initial fears had turned out to be right.

The neurologist colleague who had referred her to me was perturbed and defensive. The patient and her husband were frightened and angry. I felt humiliated as well as saddened. For me, the only saving grace was that the tumor had been inoperable from the beginning, so at least my diagnosis had not delayed potentially life-saving surgery. I told the Chetowskis how sorry I was and apologized for missing the diagnosis. I also apologized for my colleague. Mrs. Chetowski repeated that she had feared a brain tumor from the first "but after I worked through my father's suicide with you, I was sure I would be fine." Mr. Chetowski accepted my apology quietly. I offered to help her with the terminal phase of her illness, but she and her husband declined. She died two months later.

Fifteen years after her death, her son was one of four medical students assigned to my teaching service on the inpatient psychiatric unit. In his third year of medical school, he was a handsome,

41

extremely bright young man. I immediately figured out the connection as he was named for his father. I invited him to meet with me privately. I asked him if he knew I was his mother's doctor and had missed the diagnosis of her brain tumor. He said he knew. "Do you and I have any unfinished business?" I asked.

The future Dr. Chetowski paused a few seconds before answering: "I have no hard feelings toward you, doctor, but my mother's missed diagnosis and premature death were the reason I chose medicine." Pausing again he added, "I plan to become a neurosurgeon."

Reading Body Language

The ability to interpret the patient's body language and facial expressions is a valuable skill. Experienced physicians have refined this skill to a subtle art. A seasoned cardiologist senses whether a patient complaining of chest pain is suffering from heart disease or indigestion just by looking at his or her face and posture. Likewise, a good pediatrician can use similar nonverbal cues to sort out children with leukemia from those who have regressed emotionally because of an emotional challenge such as parental divorce or the arrival of a new sibling. That does not mean that these clinicians would not run appropriate tests just to make sure they have not missed something significant, but it does mean that they would have a sound idea of what they were likely to discover.

During a visit to Scott & White during the 1970s, Dr. Hans Selye, the internationally acclaimed physician who first described the physiological ramifications of stress, told me that when he was a sixteen-year-old medical student, he realized that sick people looked sick and that the sick look was remarkably similar whether they suffered from infection, cancer, cardiovascular disease, or mental illness. That observation was what had led him to devote his professional life to the study of the impact of stress on the human body.

I believe what patients need is someone skilled in the art and science of medicine and, additionally, someone to take time to listen and to understand. The Hippocratic Oath I took enjoined me to "First, do no harm." Few people have ever been harmed by being listened to and understood. Sometimes, though, doctors aren't prepared for listening. For example, during her annual physical Marjie brought up her worry over her mother's diagnosis of lymphoma. As she shared her sense of helplessness and grief with her internist, she began to cry. She reached into what looked like a box of tissue but came up with a rubber glove instead. She and her doctor started laughing. Unfortunately, Marjie's internist wasn't alone in not having tissue available for patients who explore the emotional stress underlying their physical symptoms. Many physicians are uncomfortable with this "touchy-feely" side of medicine. "Leave that to the psychiatrists," they say. "That's their specialty. None of us can know everything." The internist might say, "I know the vascular system. That's my training. That's my comfort zone."

However, except in rare cases, I observed that patients without obvious psychological pathology did not go to see a psychiatrist. If anxiety made a man's heart race, he saw his cardiologist. If stress gave a woman acid reflux, she made an appointment with her gastroenterologist. I believe health-care professionals regardless of their specialty need a basic understanding of the role of the emotions in illness and health. If a man came into an orthopedist's office saying that he had suffered from lower back pain for the past two years, nothing could be easier or more logical than to ask, "Did anything special happen two years ago?"

Often, something significant did: "I blew up when my sixteen-year-old came home with a big tattoo on his arm," one man said, "and I ordered him out of the house. My wife thought I'd gone way too far. In fact, she stood up for the kid. Our marriage has been all downhill from there."

The next question the orthopedist might ask is, "What does the back pain keep you from doing?" In the case of the patient above, it was, "It's kept me from having sex with my wife."

I learned that many times all it takes to resolve such repressed conflicting emotions and vague but life-limiting problems is for me to ask questions and listen as the patient responds, absorbing what the patient says about these formerly repressed feelings.

Doing so does not take specialized psychological training, but it does take time. Even doctors who have honed the art of medicine feel relieved when a patient comes in with a complaint that has an obvious physical cause and an equally obvious solution. "Dear God, please let this patient have gallstones" was a prayer my father and many of his Mayo Clinic colleagues offered up when they entered an examining room. Patients with gallstones emerged from treatment grateful and happy. Their painful symptom was caused by a problem that had a straightforward surgical solution. There was Mrs. Green, resting comfortably in bed surrounded by her supportive family, all admiring the bottle full of gallstones that her surgeon had given to her as a souvenir. She was the perfect patient.

But that prayer was seldom answered. Even when the referring general practitioners had a deep understanding of their patients, many of those they sent to Mayo specialists were subsequently diagnosed as CNE (Chronic Nervous Exhaustion) or the less respectful abbreviation PPP (Piss Poor Protoplasm). Gallstones, a broken leg, or any other obvious traumatic injury or illness require direct intervention. But for nine out of ten patients who came into my office with less obvious symptoms, the time-honored approach, beginning with attentive, compassionate listening, would resolve the complaint.

Medical Tests or Listening Therapy?

Patients can be harmed by what too often is today's approach of choice—expensive tests, high-tech medical procedures, and medications. Not only can these be bad for the patient, but the costly medical procedures and tests are bankrupting our healthcare system.

A prime example is what has become known as bariatric medicine, the surgical treatment of obesity. The United States is experiencing an epidemic of obesity along with its many complications, including diabetes, heart ailments, and joint disease. Clearly, being significantly overweight is not just damaging to self-esteem;

it is a serious health hazard. Despite the tummy tuck and capacity-reducing banding, patients will often gain back their excess weight. Others may lose scores of pounds but experience severe emotional distress. At its root obesity is a disorder of our relationships to food, exercise, and the significant people in our lives. Just as fat provides insulation literally, it also provides figurative insulation against emotional conflict. Another example is chemical dependency, a common complaint that often has underlying emotional causes. A diagnosis of addiction can be significant, but it is never the whole story. Alcohol and other psychoactive drugs are common tools the human psyche uses to keep conflict repressed.

Interestingly, by the way, people in the helping professions, such as doctors, teachers, and clergy, are at particular risk for becoming chemically dependent as often they struggle to solve their own conflicts by helping others with theirs. When I entered my psychiatric residency, I discovered that the Mayo Clinic offered free medical care to men and women of the cloth, wherever they served in the world. Understandably, many priests, rabbis, ministers, and nuns availed themselves of this opportunity. One outgrowth of this policy was our identification of a psychiatric disorder we came to call the "Catholic Priest Syndrome."

Our Catholic psychiatrist saw scores of Catholic priests with this pattern of dysfunction: horrible relationships with their fathers and conflicts with their sexual orientation. They escaped first through "marrying the church" and then when that began to fail them, through depression that they attempted to drown in alcohol. The term "Catholic Priest Syndrome" may not have appeared in the *Diagnostic and Statistical Manual*, the American Psychiatric Association's tome of officially recognized mental illnesses, but it was real all the same. When a physician decided that a priest required a psychiatric consultation, the interchange went something like this:

> *Gastroenterologist:* Father, your physical exam shows nothing abnormal other than mild hypertension. Your laboratory tests are all normal except for elevations in some of your liver function tests. By your history, you unquestionably are suffering from irritable bowel syndrome,

but none of the GI studies reflect any serious disease. I think you may be drinking too much, and I sense that you are depressed. I'd like you to see a psychiatrist.

Priest: I was afraid of that, but I suppose you're right. Confession is said to be good for the soul. Do you have a Roman Catholic psychiatrist?

Gastroenterologist: Yes. Dr. Maurice Barry is Catholic. I'll arrange a consultation for you.

To help maintain the patient's comfort level, Maury Berry would come to the office of the gastroenterologist for an "off the psychiatric floor" consultation. He saw a lot of priests, and he noticed that most of the therapist-patient dynamics followed a remarkably similar pattern.

Dr. Barry: Good to meet you, Father. I'm Dr. Barry from the psychiatry department.

Priest: Nice to meet you. I told Dr. Burke that confession was good for the soul. He said he thought I was drinking too much and that I was depressed. He thought you might be able to help.

Dr. Barry: Tell me about your drinking and depression.

Priest: For the past eighteen months, I've increased my drinking to over a pint of whiskey a day—after my last Mass on Sunday, maybe more. I guess I thought it would help my depression, help me sleep, help me relax.

Dr. Barry: What happened eighteen months ago?

Priest: It's hard for me to talk about it, and I haven't confessed it. A year and a half ago, my housekeeper said I'd made her pregnant. I found myself advising her to have an abortion. Imagine that! She said she'd rather commit suicide.

Dr. Barry: Did you have a long history of breaking your vows?

Priest: No, it was the first time.

Dr. Barry: And you're fifty-seven years old. How do you explain this change in your behavior?

Priest: The next part is really going to be difficult. Father Arthur and I have discussed the potential of our friendship becoming sexual. Perhaps my heterosexual experience prevented the emergence of my homosexuality.

Dr. Barry: How long have you known you were homosexual?

Priest: All my life. My father was a brutal alcoholic and had married my mother when she told him she was pregnant with me. I hated him, and I hated my mother for not protecting me from him. I turned to the church. I married God. (Begins sobbing) But, Dr. Barry, now I find that I hate God, and I'm becoming just like my father.

It would have been very simple for Maury to see the priest for a few minutes, make the dual diagnosis of major depression and alcohol dependence, and refer him to an inpatient alcohol rehabilitation program. If the depression persisted after the twenty-eight days of rehab, he could have prescribed an anti-depressant such as Elavil. But Maury had the luxury of time and truly wanted to help the priest understand the conflict that was tearing him apart, to help him obtain insight, and to do the hard demanding work, so he referred the priest, and priests with similar complaints, to Mayo's psychiatric unit for alcohol detox and intensive inpatient psychotherapy.

Anti-depressants might have been absolutely the wrong thing for Maury Barry's patients. Elavil and other anti-depressants available in the 1970s and still used today can be deadly in the hands of a suicidal individual. And a surprising number of priests commit suicide, despite the church's stern injunction that it will damn them for eternity.

When I was teaching residents, I always stressed the need to understand the interlocking relationship between repressed emotions and physical problems. Dr. Henry Maudsley, a famous nineteenth-century British pychiatrist, noted, "The sorrow that has no vent in tears may make other organs weep." I learned to review skeptically one common notation on a patient's chart "Family History Negative" (FHN). That usually meant "no close relatives with heart disease, or diabetes." But what about all the other family history, all the complex, fascinating family patterns and interactions, longings, and betrayals? These were not "negative." What about Uncle Harry's drunken car wrecks or Aunt Elena's traumatic escape from Hungary to flee the Russians? All great novels explore the convolutions of family histories. Why not medicine?

A Scott & White gastroenterologist referred Martha Felder, an intelligent fifty-one-year-old woman, to the psychiatric department. In the previous two years alone she had spent half a million dollars consulting teams of physicians in five different medical centers. Her abdomen bore scars from seven major surgeries. "My belly looks like an old golf ball," she said.

47

Mrs. Felder had come to the clinic complaining of intractable lower abdominal pain that had been plaguing her for eleven years. Despite the severity of her pain, she owned and ran a very successful gift shop. She managed to function by taking the pain medication Demerol, and she had become increasingly concerned about her dependency on this narcotic. Dozens of doctors had examined her before the gastroenterologist urged her to see me. He thought a psychiatrist would be better able to sort out the competing issues of addiction and pain management.

Along with a detailed list of the procedures she had undergone, Mrs. Felder's chart contained a telltale notation, FHN, that meant that none of the doctors had asked her the most important questions. I began by asking Mrs. Felder how long she had been in pain. "Eleven years," she replied. When I asked if anything out of the ordinary had happened eleven years earlier, she began to sob. Finally, she blurted out that her eighteen-year-old son had committed suicide by shooting himself in the belly with a ten-gauge shotgun.

I told Mrs. Felder that I thought we could resolve her symptoms and help heal her grief. She agreed to be admitted to Scott & White's inpatient psychiatric unit. Withdrawing her from Demerol took a little more than a week. Meanwhile, her work in individual and group therapy brought about significant breakthroughs. After ten days we dismissed her from the hospital. She returned for two follow-up visits, and by then her pain had disappeared completely.

To Test or Not to Test

Even though they care deeply for their patients, good physicians often run the risk of dangerous overtesting, overmedicating, and ordering unnecessary surgery. The best way for me to avoid doing that was to listen intently to the patient and try to recognize repressed conflicts. Recognizing the role of repressed conflict in the formation of symptoms and knowing the history of the behavioral patterns of my patients and my patients' families helped me ask the right questions and tailor the treatment.

Today's technology puts powerful tools at our disposal; however, sometimes physicians interpret availability as obligation.
Fear of professional embarrassment creates another strong impe-
tus to overtest and overtreat. Consider the chagrin of overhearing
a colleague say of you in the doctors' lounge, "Looks like Jones
missed that lesion. Should have been obvious." Not to mention
the distress of having to admit to patients and their families that
you didn't pick up that blood clot in the leg or that tiny spot on
the mammogram. The threat of malpractice suits is omnipresent,
and while the system was developed to address the very real and
serious consequences of incompetence or impairment, it exerts
pressure to run one more test, the latest, most expensive assay, on
the principle of CYA (Cover Your Ass).

But defensive medicine can never be efficient medicine. Testing before listening is too expensive. Rather than trying one high-
tech tool after another, I found it more effective and less potentially harmful to balance the patient's needs with the economics
of medicine and to employ the time-tested art of listening first,
and calling for expensive scans and exploratory surgeries only
when listening failed.

Hysterics are patients at particular risk of being caught up in an
expensive yet probably futile medical maelstrom. Freud brought
hysteria to popular awareness by describing dramatic symptoms
prevalent among the Victorian bourgeoisie, such as unexplained
blindness, deafness, paralysis, and seizures, and by explaining
how they resulted from repressed sexual impulses. Hysteria is still
with us, but its physical expression has changed, as has the nature
of the emotions repressed. The woman referred to Freud because
she was struck blind on seeing her father having sex with her
nanny has been replaced by the woman whose chronic abdominal
pain prevents her from having sex with her unfaithful husband.
Hysterical conversion is quite common. Even specialists such as
orthopedists and cardiologists say that their schedules are full of
patients whose chief complaints are confusing. A fractured femur
is obvious, as is a leaky heart valve. The doctor can see and feel
the former and hear the latter. But for every one of those, the
orthopedist sees nine wrenched backs or bad knees, and the cardi-

49

ologist sees cases of rapid heartbeat, anxiety or chest pain which are likely to be cases of hysterical conversion.

Hypochondriasis

Sometimes hysteria comes packaged with hypochondriasis. Confronted with hypochondriasis and hysteria, specialists run tests to ferret out the cause. When the tests come back negative, as they so often do, the doctor often orders more. And when the last, most exacting, most expensive, state-of-the-art scan shows nothing, physicians have a term for the syndrome. "That patient," they say, seldom bothering to conceal their anger and frustration, "is a crock."

"Crock" is slang for hypochondriac. Unlike malingerers (those who pretend an incapacity), hypochondriacs genuinely believe they are seriously ill, but like malingerers they are very hard to treat. They often present with a mysterious, rare disease, and they seek out doctor after doctor, all of whom cannot find a physical problem. Nonetheless, hypochondriacs assert their conviction that something must be wrong. For me, these patients were easy to spot. They showed up for their first appointments bearing a thick file of test results. It was not uncommon for hypochondriacs to have had multiple surgeries and invasive tests and to have been prescribed so many drugs that they brought their medicines to the office in a shoe box. Each subsequent test had left the patient more invested in the symptom, more certain that he or she had something serious. "After all," they said, "why else would these doctors be going to all this trouble and expense?"

No one raises the anger of physicians more than hypochondriacs. Marjie and I produced a film in which we portrayed the interaction between a crock and her doctor. The film was called *Hypochondriasis and Healthcare: A Tug of War,* and it won a 1978 Golden Cine Award for best medical documentary. We screened it at numerous professional conferences where we did our best to create a nonjudgmental environment, giving doctors a forum for venting their heretofore repressed feelings about hypochondriacal patients.

50

Sometimes, rather than playing the film, we enacted the scenario live. After one of these performances, a middle-aged physician jumped up from the audience, pointed his finger at me angrily and shouted, "Whatever you do, don't leave that patient here in St. Louis!" Clearly, he could not tolerate his city's having one more hypochondriac. Marjie said later that his angry outburst was the best compliment she had ever received for her acting.

I soon learned that hypochondriacs would never get well. In their life experience they have never been well. These demanding, frustrating patients are extreme and vivid examples of individuals whose repressed emotions have caused debilitating physical symptoms. When I understood this dynamic I was much less subject to frustration and anger.

A version of the question I posed to every patient referred to me with a physical complaint helped me sort out the hypochondriacs from those in whom a specific repressed emotional conflict had manifested itself as a physical problem. When a patient complained of fatigue, pain in a number of organs, nausea, or another diffuse chronic symptom I asked, "When was the last time you felt well in every way?" If the response was "Two Christmases ago," I'd follow with "And what happened two Christmases ago?" encouraging a story that began with "Two Christmases ago." Then I knew this was not likely a hypochondriacal patient.

On the other hand, a hypochondriac would always answer, "Doctor, I've never been well." For these individuals the story began, "My mother was sick during the entire pregnancy. The obstetrician said it was the most difficult delivery," and so on. Hypochondriacs recounted harrowing childhood illnesses such as brucellosis, typhoid fever, or malaria ("the only case ever reported in Iowa"). They bragged about these ailments as if they were badges of distinction. The more serious and exotic the disease, the prouder they were.

Hypochondrical women recounted the horrors of their menarche (beginning their menstrual cycle): so severe that they required trips to the emergency room for shots of narcotics. Often a woman would recall her early painful periods as the only time she felt close to her mother, who massaged her back, fed her choco-

51

late pudding, and comforted her. She hoped I would duplicate her mother's comforting, which, of course, I could not do. Hysterectomies were often performed to "cure" this problem, but the same terrible pain would occur elsewhere in the abdomen or in the lower back, usually on a monthly basis.

In hypochondriacs, the real underlying need is for nurturing, not the fatigue, the aches, or the rare cancer, or exotic infection they beg the doctor to find and explain. What a hypochondriac unconsciously craves from his or her physician is not a cure, but attention. When I put aside the compelling desire to fix what was essentially unfixable, I could provide treatment safely by educating my patients about hypochondriasis and enlisting their cooperation in managing their condition.

I told hypochondriacs that they had a serious, often disabling illness and that I would be willing to help them obtain Social Security medical disability. I stressed that they needed medical care, but that it had to be with the expectation that they would never feel entirely well. The goal of the care would be to protect them from harmful (even fatal) tests, procedures, surgeries, and medications that had no possibility of doing them any good. I told them that, in my experience, and in that of most other physicians, every new test, procedure, medication, or surgery helps for about three months. Then the effect wears off.

After that part of the conversation with a hypochondriac, I described the treatment plan. I would see these patients on a regular basis, once or twice a month, to evaluate and respond to their complaints, but I would limit the number of drugs, tests, surgeries, and other procedures. "You're addicted to these things," I would explain, "and there won't be many more of them." Those who could not accept this approach left in search of yet another physician who would prescribe another round of costly and often dangerous interventions. But many patients accepted my prescription, and we developed long-term therapeutic relationships. Although they never got well, they were out of danger.

This phenomenon extends even to pet owners and their pets. Dr. Gary Gosney, a small-animal veterinarian, tells about his experience with hypochondrical pet owners who will project their symptoms onto their pets and request treatment for their pet such as a hysterectomy. He further noticed that any procedure he performed provided relief for the owner for about three months.

Hypochondriacs may well be the most vulnerable of patients, at risk for being harmed or even killed, all in the name of healing by a system armed and ready to attack acute infections, treat traumatic injuries, save people from such life-threatening diseases as cancer, and manage chronic ailments like diabetes. Of course, hypochondriacs are vulnerable to the same acute and chronic diseases as the rest of us, and I always tried to be alert to a marked change in the patient's pattern, in case there were, in fact, a physical ailment.

There are several other diagnoses that never respond well to insight therapy. Malingerers, for example, are genuine fakes. They consciously mimic symptoms for obvious gain. A woman seeking a hefty settlement for disabling neck and shoulder pain may sue the driver of a car that bumped hers at a stoplight. In court the plaintiff may claim that as a result of this fender-bender, she suffers chronic pain that prevents her from lifting her arms. Sitting in the witness stand, she demonstrates for the judge and the jury that she cannot raise her arms above her shoulders. Understandably, she becomes furious when the defense counsel plays a videotape showing her hanging potted plants on her porch. Also Munchausen's Syndrome, a rare form of malingering in which people consciously injure themselves in order to be admitted to the hospital, does not respond well to treatment. For example, one of my father's diabetic patients repeatedly overdosed with insulin, resulting in her hospitalization and tests for a possible tumor of the pancreas. My dad suspected Munchausen's, and because she was in the hospital, he could tag her insulin with radioactive iodine so the next time the patient tried her ploy, the evidence would show up on a test. And it did.

Distressed people turn first to doctors other than psychiatrists because it is less frightening to hear that they have something wrong physically, even a life-threatening condition, than it is to hear that they have to confront a long-buried and heavily defended emotional pain that lies at the root of their vague, chronic,

53

non-specific symptoms. The same holds true for many physicians. They seem far more comfortable treating a challenging physical pathology than they are even touching emotional conflict.

Patients who came to our clinic shared one fear, usually unconscious: "Am I dying?" Their doctors back home had been stumped by their cases and had sent them to an American equivalent of Lourdes for a miracle cure. A sophisticated team was bound to identify something truly awful. If, as was usually the case, the team found nothing out of the ordinary, perhaps nothing at all, it could be even scarier for the patient than a serious diagnosis. "Are you sure you haven't missed anything?" the frightened patient might insist. "Aren't there any other tests?" One hypochondriac man begged, "I've been everywhere, to every medical center, but no one has found the problem. There must be a way to find it! Please open me up and see. Then I'll know what's wrong with me. I wouldn't mind even a touch of cancer."

Somatization

One of my major challenges was persuading patients who had come to Scott & White complaining of, say, stomach pain, that the symptoms were not imaginary. "Are you saying it's all in my head?" a patient might cry out. Somatization, the expression of emotional distress as physical distress and sometimes disease, is one of the most serious issues in psychiatry, in fact, in all of medicine. Grief over the loss of a loved one, for example, can suppress the immune system, leaving a widow or widower open to everything from infected shaving nicks to cancer. Stress can throw a diabetic's blood sugar out of control, and untreated depression can put a patient at risk for heart disease. The actual problem is almost always complicated by an underlying emotional conflict.

Often patients came to my office at Scott & White angry with their doctors for having referred them to a psychiatrist. My mentor, Howard Rome, taught me a method for introducing the psychological roots of physical complaints through a demonstration involving clenching fists. I used the method he taught me many times, as with one patient who said, "Doctor, I can't understand

54

how some inner stress could cause this pain."

"Show me your hand." I said. "It looks like a normal hand. Is it causing you any pain?"

"No."

"We could do a complete examination of all the nerves, bones, and blood vessels and find nothing wrong. Make a fist. Good. Make it tighter. Tighter again. Make it as tight as you can."

The patient, seeming a bit puzzled, did so, and I said, "If you keep your fist tight like that hour after hour, day after day, week after week, what's it going to do?"

The patient answered, "It's going to cramp and hurt. It's doing that already."

"Your pain is caused by your tensing. Now, what's causing the tension in your life?"

I've had many such conversations, and with the release of their clenched fists, the patients almost always began describing some distressing situation or conflict that coincided with the onset of the symptoms. For most the first step to insight was understanding that the symptom was not the illness, that the chief complaint might not have been the real problem.

For example, Mr. Ellis, an incredibly handsome man in his late fifties, had been incapacitated by back pain for six months. He had undergone a number of orthopedic evaluations in Dallas without a diagnosis or an effective treatment. When he entered my office, I was enormously impressed by his appearance and charm. He looked like someone had gone to Central Casting to find the perfect CEO. He had, in fact, become the CEO of a large Dallas company eight months before coming to the clinic, but he said his incapacitating back pain had caused him to spend most days in bed.

His history revealed that he had come from a large family. He was the youngest child of seven and had never experienced any emotional problems. His family lived next to a country club, and he worked for the golf pro through high school. He starred on the golf team in high school and earned a full scholarship to Southern Methodist University in Dallas where he joined a Greek fraternity and took the golf team to several championships. He gave thought

55

to turning pro when one of his fraternity brothers, whose father was the CEO of a major corporation, persuaded him to join his father's organization. His golf ability and appearance allowed a meteoric rise in the company, and he became the executive vice-president, second in command. "While I was extremely popular, I had to rely on my boss for critical decisions, and when he died eight months ago, I felt lost," he said.

Mr. Ellis had trouble understanding the dynamics of his pain and his repressed emotional conflict. So I did the clenched fist demonstration with him. As his clenched fist relaxed, tears began to flow, and he said he'd had enormous tension all his life "because I knew, deep down, that I didn't have the intelligence to manage responsibility. I barely got through college." He dreaded being in charge of his company, and the feeling of being lost translated into his back pain which caused him to regress to his bed. Psychometric testing revealed he had an IQ of eighty. (Average IQ is one hundred.) When we discussed the cause of his pain being related to his inability to function in his new position, he was relieved and said, "I need to take early retirement."

In listening and hearing and asking probing questions, I had success in leading patients to the kind of self-revelation that is called true insight. That is, they came to terms with themselves and their real history and their real lives.

Chapter Five
Diagnosing

Repression as Survival

Repression is the mechanism by which emotional conflict which cannot be faced at the time it occurs is forcefully submerged from the conscious mind into the unconscious. Repression starts out as an essential survival mechanism. When I began practicing psychiatry in the late 1950s, I developed an efficient method of psychotherapy. My patients typically saw some positive results after the first visit and resolved their major problems within two to three months of hour-long once-a-week sessions. I found that the most effective approach was to help them gain insight into the experiences underlying their distress, the ones they had repressed.

The mind has ingenious but ultimately damaging ways of protecting people from these memories. Young children, for example, are totally dependent on their parents and lack the skills to assert themselves, so when a man sexually abuses his eight-year-old stepdaughter, and her mother rejects her pleas to intervene, the little girl's psyche buries the entire experience. This allows her to remain in the family, which she relies on for food, shelter, and security. Keeping the traumatic memory below the level of conscious awareness protects her when she is most vulnerable.

Of course, it would be better if some wise and perceptive adult like a teacher, a relative, a pediatrician, or a minister spotted the signs of abuse and acted to protect the child, but children and other vulnerable individuals have never been able to count on such help. Our psychological defenses evolved over the millennia to allow us to survive when assistance was not forthcoming. However, repression exacts a steep toll. It saps energy, creates physical symptoms, and inhibits our ability to trust and be close to others in mutually life-enhancing relationships. It also blocks what Dr. Mikhaili Csikszentmihalyi, former chair of the Department of Psychology at the University of Chicago, calls the sense of joy

57

and transcendence that fuels creativity and life's other meaningful pleasures—"flow." By the time a person reaches adulthood, repression has almost always outlived its usefulness. Adults have the life skills, emotional maturity, and other resources to face the traumatic truth, but their psyches continue to keep this repressed material locked tightly out of sight. "Danger! Do not enter! Top Secret."

A five year-old child who sees a parent murdered cannot cope. But once the person's ego is stronger, say, when the child's reaches the age of thirty, the damage caused by the mechanism of repression outweighs its protective value. By bringing the patient's memory to the surface, then guiding him or her through the grief, fear, and guilt surrounding that circumstance, I could often relieve the distress. The greater the inner conflict, the more difficult it is to transcend. The worse the emotional traffic congestion, the harder it is to get to "flow." Conversely, resolving inner conflict clears the road to such flow.

Often my patients found it extremely difficult to tell the people trying to help them what their underlying problem was. Until they broke through that stoutly constructed barrier, they could not know what it concealed because repression works. It keeps the cause of the distress from becoming conscious. Unless that cause is unearthed, it stays buried and continues to result in a host of symptoms, and unfortunately, those buried causes can continue to induce pain not just on one generation but on more than one.

Dr. Roy Smythe, the head of the Department of Surgery at Scott & White, captures that reality in this quote from a novel he is writing:

> There are millions of events and decisions in a life, some random, others volitional, some in parallel, some in series. The vast majority of things we think and decide and act on are like debris in the water, insignificant, having no bearing on the future state, predicting nothing. Most are cast off to the riverbank, trapped in the foamy eddy currents or in the reeds, floating for a period of time, and then falling beneath the water. In the collective life of every family, however, are linked occurrences; the ones that determine what comes next, and what will likely come after that. They coalesce in the middle of the river of a family's life, lining up in the current, becoming for some the current itself.

Understanding the existence of this current has been a main force of my psychotherapy. In fact, my psychiatric practice had three fundamental characteristics. It was insight-oriented, goal-directed, and short-term.

Insight-oriented, Goal-directed, Short-term Therapy

In psychotherapy, "insight" occurs when repressed, unconscious material becomes fully conscious on the gut level. At this "Eureka!" moment, the working-through often unravels the emotional knot and allows the patient to feel the thrill of transcending conflict to discover unity (the oneness of being). This form of insight should not be confused with a person's reaching a rational understanding of the root of a problem. It is experiential, as opposed to intellectual. When a patient was able to say, "My stepfather abused me sexually, and my mother blamed me for it, so she treated me as a rival instead of defending me," she identified the root of her anxiety, depression, and abdominal pain. But I knew that only re-experiencing that sense of betrayal, anger, and shame would resolve her problems.

Insight-oriented therapy required the patient and I work together to bring to the surface the repressed memories and conflicts that produced their problems. During every first session, I explained that we would have a contract and that each of us must agree to hold up our end of the bargain no matter how much resistance we experienced in relation to dealing with whatever was repressed. We traded home and work phone numbers and agreed that we would keep our appointments unless we could explain the reason for canceling or changing. Although I had one patient who drove twelve hundred miles round-trip every week in her Volkswagen, I generally shied away from outpatients who lived more than an hour away since resistance to psychotherapy was so significant. Distance was too easy an excuse to cancel an appointment.

Goal-directed therapy was the second major characteristic of my approach to healing patients. At the beginning of therapy, the patient and I agreed on the specific outcome we wanted to achieve. The patient had to state the goal in a positive way so he or she could collaborate with me. "Every time I'm about to succeed, I do something to insure failure and I want to stop doing that" is positive and would be a workable goal, whereas, "I'm unhappy and overweight and I want to change that" is a negative complaint that would not be workable. Another example of a workable goal is "I want to be able to finish my work so I don't lose my job." The negative of that might be "I'm afraid of being fired, and I don't want that to happen." When children are young, they are sometimes unwilling to go to second base without taking first base with them, but in order for a patient to achieve her goal, she had to be willing to risk safety, leave first base behind and set her sights on home base.

During the course of therapy, the goal could change, but the change had to be mutually agreed upon. Without a goal I could not identify the source of resistance. With a goal I could say, "You're silent today. What's keeping you from working toward your goal?" In the first hour, we discussed the difference between therapeutic help and dependency gratification. I explained that if the patient just wanted to have me around as a paid friend to give nonjudgmental support, he or she had come to the wrong place.

The third characteristic of my practice was to limit the therapy to a short term. To accelerate the therapeutic process I used techniques that broke through the conscious level to reach deep into the unconscious. Some of these were novel. Others, such as hypnosis, were not. Some techniques followed the same route that artists use to access their creativity. Patients wrote poetry, carved figures, made self-portraits, did abstract drawings of dreams, and painted their current families, and families of origin. Even examining family photos could be powerfully illuminating. All of these methods helped me bypass the normal verbal and intellectual resistance to psychotherapy.

Chapter Six
Working Toward a Breakthrough

The Arts as Therapy

For my fifty-fifth birthday, I received an exceptional gift. I'd been carving on everything from soap to wood as long as I can remember, but I had never really studied the techniques of stone sculpting. The present was a six-week stone sculpture class at the Elizabet Ney Museum in Austin, Texas, and by the time I finished the last class, I knew I needed to know more.

I'd been told by one of my classmates about an American-born sculptor, Jon Fisher, who lived and worked in Pietra Santa, Italy. She said the sculptor and his buddies met at the Igea Bar every night at five, and that if I just showed up, he would find me a place to stay and help me buy the marble and tools I needed to help me become a real sculptor. I'm usually a very organized traveler. I know who will meet me, where I'll stay, and what I'll do each day, but my trip to Italy was totally different.

I flew to Milan, caught a train, and landed in Pietra Santa at about four in the afternoon. I got off the train and walked the block from the station to the town square. Before I could find someone to ask how to get to the Igea Bar, I spotted the sign. The door was open, but when I walked in I saw only two customers. The bartender motioned for me to come get a drink, but I waved him off indicating I was meeting someone and wanted to wait by the door. At five minutes after five o'clock four men sauntered into the bar, and without even noticing me, went to a table I assumed was where they always sat. I was so nervous about being in a foreign country, not speaking the language, and not having secured a place to stay that night that I just bolted over to them and asked if one of them was Jon Fisher. A long-haired, bearded, dusty, forty year-old man claimed the name. He turned out to be everything I'd been told and more. After we all got to know each other a bit, Jon got me settled in at a small hotel across the street from the bar and said he'd pick me up the next morning.

The next day we went shopping for tools, and when I had purchased everything I needed, we went to his studio. Jon talked to me while he worked on a magnificent larger-than-life figure. I stood in awe until he stopped and said it was time for me to start on my own piece. He led me to a table where he had placed a medium-sized chunk of marble. As he walked away he said, "This piece of marble is from a vein that Michelangelo quarried for his work five hundred years ago."

I laid out all my tools, brushed off the marble, went to the bathroom, talked to one of the other sculptors on my way back from the bathroom, tied a bandana around my head, reorganized my tools, and brushed off the marble. I had no idea where to begin.

Then Jon, recognizing my reluctance to make a mark, broke the silence and said, "Remember when you were a child and you'd lie on your back and look at the clouds, and the longer you looked the more shapes you saw, like giant rabbits, humpback whales, or sailing ships? Now look at this piece of stone as if it were a cloud. Start chiseling away at the marble and see what emerges. Just begin, and keep chiseling until you see the sculpture that is trying to emerge. The sculpture is already there. You just have to remove the excess marble around it."

As a sculptor I was to look until I "saw." The idea was certainly not foreign to me. As a psychiatrist I had learned to listen until I "heard." One of the most effective methods I used to help patients uncover repressed emotional conflicts and to express their feelings was art therapy. In a sense, through creative art efforts, patients chiseled away at their own "marble" of repression and were able to discover themselves and heal.

My mother was a talented woman who wanted desperately for me to find an artistic niche for myself in the world. Perhaps that's why I found art to be so effective in helping patients mine their unconscious. When I was a small child, my mother taught me how to sculpt animals from bars of soap. I can't remember when I did not draw and doodle. Even during the hectic days and nights of medical school and residency, I carved blocks of wood. As I created these pictures and objects, I always sensed that I was bypassing the part of my mind that mastered chemical formulas and memorized the names of muscles. Things would appear in my art that had nothing to do with intellectual processing. Yet they were mine. Clearly, they came from emotions and experiences that were hidden from my rational mind.

I make masks from clay, I do serigraphs, and I sculpt stone. My sculptures have grown from small figurative pieces to larger-than-life statues. Art is not a hobby to me. It is an essential part of my life, integral to who I am. After my father's death in 1987, my mother made her last trip to Texas. She arrived in late March because she loved our field of bluebonnets. In my usual carving place underneath the live oak trees with shade and a breeze, I was finishing a green soapstone frog to give to her. I told her the frog was a symbol of health and healing. She smiled and thanked me. Then she said, "Bob, dear, I want to tell you something." A feeling inside me commanded that I remain quiet and listen to her. She told me how much she loved me, how she hoped that my involvement with art was in part because of her encouragement, and that she was proud I had shared my creative spirit with so many people. After a few moments she said, "Watching you create something for me, floods me with the warm memory I have of the closeness I felt with my father when he allowed me to sit next to him, turning the pages, while he played his Steinway piano for Enrico Caruso's concert in 1915. I was eight years old. That beautiful music transcended the union with me, my father, Caruso, and the several thousand people in the Pittsburgh Concert Hall." I remained quiet and accepted her gift.

Just as space for creativity was a must for my home, I considered it essential for the psychiatric unit. The main clinic building was completed a few months after I joined Scott & White. The new space liberated me from my temporary digs (the former Ear, Nose, and Throat Lab). The building was the first site designated for the psychiatry department, but it contained little space for group therapy, let alone creative activities. Lodged on the fifth floor of an octagonal tower, Psychiatry had the same layout as Surgery and Cardiology. We all had wedge-shaped patient rooms arrayed around a central nurses' station for keeping an eye on heart monitors and respiration rates. This cluster design represented a significant improvement over the long, straight corridors of traditional inpatient units, but it was unsuitable for even conventional psychiatric care, let alone any kind of innovative approach.

When I started our department, Occupational Therapy was the mainstay of inpatient psychiatric programs nationwide. It featured such craft-kit projects as beaded leather moccasins and enameled ashtrays. The goal was to get patients out of their rooms and interacting socially. I did not have much faith in the appropriateness of this approach. Personally, when I was troubled I wanted to be alone creating something genuinely expressive, not trying to interact with other people and engaging in busy work.

So for two years I rented a church bus several afternoons a week and sent our sixteen patients to the studio of local artist Forrest Gist, a former West Texas oilfield roughneck with a degree in advertising, art and design, and a man with a mustache like a Western movie sheriff's. At Forrest's studio, these severely emotionally ill people would spend three hours attacking large stretched canvases with big brushes and lots of colorful acrylic paint. Then he loaded up the afternoon's work and took it back to Scott & White so the patients could discuss their creations with their doctors.

The 1970s were a Golden Age for medicine. Medicare had recently been put into effect insuring every American over sixty-five and many others with disabilities. Most industries were still unionized, and unions negotiated generous health insurance plans for their members. Insurance companies, for their part, placed few limits on coverage because they could afford to do that. The treatment options available in those days were not that expensive. The money was there for me to do whatever I felt would yield the best results for our patients. As we say in Texas, "I had me a bird's nest on the ground."

In 1973 we were offered space in the Special Treatment Center, a new annex to the main hospital. The original plan was for Psychiatry to share the building with Oncology, Endocrinology,

Orthopedics, and Physical Therapy. With a bit of political maneuvering and a lot of luck, I succeeded in securing the entire first floor for Psychiatry. I felt as if I were an artist in a white coat being handed the opportunity to design an environment for the practice and development of novel techniques in insight therapy. I was given what amounted to a blank check.

Forrest Gist worked with me to design a twenty by thirty-foot creative therapy room that most professional artists could only dream of. One of the long walls featured sliding glass doors leading to a protected grassy yard. We had our own spacious, light-filled art studio right on the unit, and the patients could go there any hour of the day or night.

Having a designated place for art helped our patients overcome the natural resistance to beginning a creative project. Even professional writers and artists frequently find themselves compulsively cleaning their workspace, making grocery lists, and weeding the garden—anything to put off making a mark. But once started, the creative process flows, inner resistance disappears, and time vanishes. Both Freud and Jung believed that although the unconscious can be a negative force, it also contains positive energy that can fuel creativity and lead to transcendence.

Ours was not the first program to use art therapy. It had been employed in European and American psychiatric hospitals since the early twentieth century. By the 1960s art therapists had established themselves as a profession. A number of university psychology departments around the country offered advanced degrees in this increasingly structured discipline. An art therapist became part of the treatment team, involved in morning rounds, reviewing diagnoses and treatment plans, and charting his or her observations. As the patient worked away, many art therapists would comment on the brush strokes and discuss the significance of colors saying things like, "Why don't you try using warmer colors here?" In hospitals employing this approach, there was always a lot of chatter in the activity room.

However, at Scott & White we approached art and therapy in a very different, perhaps unique, way. In our unit the room was almost always silent as the creativity flowed. Often the only

65

sound was the soft whisk-whisk of brushes. You could hear people breathe, even hear a push-pin drop. Forrest was there to give advice, and he was asked questions like, "How do I mix a really bright green?" but he did not offer interpretations or suggestions, apart from urging cranky Central Texas ranchers to "Make a mark! Make a mess!" Forrest was an artist, not an art therapist. He never contributed to or even saw a patient's chart. On admission our patients were shown the studio and told they could use it whenever they wanted to paint their symptoms, dreams, and self-portraits, or just to experiment with the materials. We explained that a professional artist would be there for three hours a day to answer any questions they might have about technique.

On their first visit to the studio, Forrest showed patients the materials, which were simple: art board, thick brushes, jars of acrylic paint, and buckets of fat crayons. The brushes were large, we explained, because we did not want detail. When the patient resisted, "I'm not an artist, I can't draw!" Forrest cleared up the mission of the program in his own West Texas way. Typically, he would say something like this:

> Now, look, this is not about turning you into a Picasso or a Rembrandt. This is not about art. It's about creativity. Creativity is the basis for art, but it doesn't work the other way around. There's a big difference. We're trying to get you to see a possibility for change. When we see people in this condition, they don't see the possibility for change. They're backed up in a corner or change is so scary they can't look at it. If you didn't feel that way, you wouldn't be here. I want you to think about the possibilities for your life. I have people tell me their kids can draw better than they can. I tell them if they'd practiced drawing as much as they'd practice writing, they'd be a lot better. Anyway, this is not about being a good artist.
>
> I'll be asking you to draw your families, yourself, your feelings, thoughts and ideas, but you'll be working in the abstract. Don't plan anything. As you translate your feelings to your painting, don't give a form to them. You see this coffee cup? It's a coffee cup because we say it is. If I put an X on a sheet of paper and tell you it is a cup, then it is a cup because I'm telling you it's a cup. If a football coach shows you a play sheet with rows of X's, you know those X's are football players. Right?
>
> So now that you know you don't have to draw "pictures," get your

66

colors and go to work. If I could teach you to be great artists, I would, but I can't. What I can do is give you these four rules of my workshop:

1. When you get yourself in too deep and you don't want to paint any more, go to the house. (Translation: Get out of the art workshop and go back to your room.) I'm not here to make your life worse. If you can't get into it, just take a hike. I don't want you in here disturbing the people who are working.

2. If your doctor prescribes medicine, stay on it.

3. Cut yourself a little slack. We're all in this shit together.

4. Don't kill yourself. If you kill yourself, we can't treat you. You're just dead. This stuff you're doing in here is the cornerstone of your existence. If you can't look at something one way and then see it another way—that's what creativity is—if you can't see the possibility of change, if you don't do that, can't see change, you won't get better.

So with Forrest Gist as the resident artist, the patients painted. Each patient painted on twenty-four by twenty-four inch fiber boards with large brushes and acrylic paints. The table top itself, (See below) after many years of splattered paint, became a work of art. Forrest never critiqued the patients' work. Some of the paintings showed sophisticated visual composition and deft brush strokes, but that was not the point. Even the clumsiest drawings offered valuable insights into long-buried conflicts. It was creative therapy, not art class.

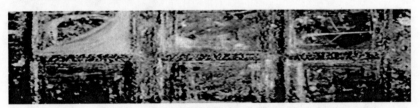

Illustration No. 1: The wooden table used by patients eventually became caked with vibrant color. It's now a wall piece in the author's home.

Expression versus Medication

The importance of patients being able to express inner conflicts as opposed to being medicated was the core of our unit's culture.

When a patient awoke in the middle of the night complaining of a terrifying dream, the nurse on duty would suggest that the patient go to the creative workshop and paint the nightmare rather than taking a sleeping pill. "If you paint it," she explained, "you can show it to the doctor in the morning." Most patients commented that they were surprised at how much they enjoyed painting. "I've never done it before!" they would exclaim. I reminded them that as little children, they could not stop making pictures on any surface available. This urge first got inhibited if their parents said something like, "Whoever marked up this wall with purple crayons is in big trouble!"

We achieved some startling breakthroughs with our form of art therapy. One in particular stands out in my memory. A retired Air Force general who had been treated unsuccessfully for depression at some of the most respected psychiatric hospitals in the world returned from an afternoon in Forrest's studio with a painting of a dark blob lodged in a tunnel. The blob struck me as an apt depiction of someone severely depressed. "There I am," the general told me, "lodged in my depression." We both looked at the painting for a while without saying anything. Then I realized the tunnel was pink—feminine. After some more silence he said excitedly, "My God! The depression is my sanctuary. I can't leave it."

That was insight. He realized his depression was his sanctuary, and he and I both knew that his depression was not the problem that needed treatment. We both knew he and his wife needed to return home where she could be in command. He had tried many antidepressants, electroshock treatments, and had even considered a prefrontal lobotomy. Through creative therapy he had come to understand that what he needed was to be nurtured and to be allowed to express his long-suppressed need to be dependent. He and his wife no longer had the expectation that they would find some drug or procedure to treat his "depression."

Another patient, Mrs. Kleinman, a middle-aged woman, came to Scott & White complaining of chronic abdominal pain and generalized fatigue. After our internists had examined her and found no physical cause for her symptoms, she was admitted to the psychiatric unit for withdrawal from the narcotic Demerol and the barbiturate Seconal. During her initial assessment she reported having experienced years of pain and despondency. She had been in psychiatric hospitals eight times. Sometimes she felt better for a while, but the symptoms always returned within a month or two.

"Nothing, even shock treatments, has helped!" she told me despairingly. "I'm ready to give up. Life isn't worth it." Mrs. Kleinman agreed to participate in our creative workshop where she produced scores of paintings. One day we were going over a painting that was a landscape depicting a road going between two hills. The sun stood low near the right horizon. When I asked her if it was rising or setting, she thought it was a setting sun. "But there's no one in the picture," she observed. Then I drew Mrs. Kleinman's attention to a small white rectangle next to the road. "Oh, I didn't see that!" she said. As she looked at the little rectangle, she began to sob uncontrollably and cried out, "It's my baby in her casket!" Then the story poured out. At age sixteen, she was seduced by a trusted uncle. She became pregnant and had a secret abortion. This was long before *Roe v. Wade*, so the procedure was both illegal and dangerous, not to mention a source of shame. She had never discussed this with anyone, not even her mother or her uncle. "It would have exploded the family," she said. "My father would have killed him."

During her eight previous hospitalizations, Mrs. Kleinman had never mentioned the seduction and abortion. But the art therapy had bypassed her well-entrenched defenses. In subsequent sessions she was able to re-experience and then resolve much of her anger and grief. When her detox was complete, she left the unit and continued psychotherapy as an outpatient.

Another patient who gained insight through art was a young woman who painted a picture of herself leaving her apartment, holding a credit card in her hand. Mimicking the then current ad campaign for American Express, the caption under the painting read, "Depression. Don't leave home without it." When she showed me the painting, I laughed and then we talked about how important her depression was. She could not tolerate the vulnerability of being emotionally close to other people, and her depression provided a shield. It kept them away. She needed it to protect her, and she would not feel safe leaving home without it. That insight helped her learn to overcome her depression enough to relate to people most of the time and to accept that she could also expect to have occasional "pajama days" when she never got dressed or left home.

In 1976, after Dr. Donald Weismann, a University of Texas professor in the arts, had visited our psychiatric unit he wrote:

> As you well know, I cannot speak with any expertise concerning the psychiatric/medical dimensions of the program. However, as I see it, the principal, logistical-plus and general value of this program involving painting is that it encourages a non-verbal means of communication and expression and introduces a third "physical presence" existing between doctor and patient. By that I mean that once the patient has formulated and presented a painting and chooses to show it, then a potentially rich and helpful conversation should be able to take place through that third physical presence or "vehicle."

Occasional Non-response to Art Therapy

Sometimes, however, such art therapy failed. I had some patients with whom I could not make progress and others whose improvement crumbled once they returned to their old environment.

Mr. Roberts was a thirty-eight-year-old man who was admitted to our psychiatry unit in 1969 after confessing to his wife that he heard voices commanding him to kill her and their two children. She told me that although he had a successful East Texas floral business, he had suffered previous psychiatric problems for which he had been prescribed medication. The complete medical and neurological evaluation I ordered came back normal. The psychological tests were consistent with borderline personality disorder. When patients with this condition are doing relatively well, they seem like reasonably well-functioning neurotics, but when they are under stress, they may develop delusions and hallucinations. Mr. Roberts' psychological history was remarkable in that he remembered an incident that had occurred when he was a toddler. His mother had told him that he was evil and should never have been born. That was consistent with his wife's description of his family as very disturbed. "It's a wonder that he survived it," she said, adding that he kept all his feelings "locked up."

I admitted Mr. Roberts to the unit and placed him on the anti-psychotic Stelazine, and the anti-depressant Parnate. In addition to participating in individual and group therapy, he spent a great deal of time in the painting workshop. Of the hundreds of paintings he produced, most featured volcanoes, tornadoes, or floods.

After two weeks with us, Mr. Roberts had improved significantly. When he said he wanted a pass to spend Easter Sunday with his family and attend church, I left it up to them. His admission had been voluntary, so he and his relatives had the final say. His wife had serious reservations about this plan, but his mother and their fundamentalist minister pressured Mrs. Roberts to grant his request, which she did. Mr. Roberts was to leave the unit Sunday morning and return that evening, but late that afternoon his wife called me at home to say that he had shot himself. "He blew his brains out at the altar," she told me over the phone. Mrs. Roberts reported that her husband had gone to see the pastor and after praying with him, the pastor had told him he was evil. "Both the pastor and my mother-in-law are crazy," Mrs. Roberts declared.

Patients with borderline personality disorder often believe they are "bad seeds." To compensate they try to be perfect and to protect their families by distancing themselves. Sometimes this takes the form of abandonment, and at other times it takes the form of suicide. Mr. Roberts' pastor and his mother reinforced his delusion that he was irredeemably evil and needed to eliminate himself in order to protect the people he loved. More often severe symptoms are the "guard dogs" trying to keep the conflicts in the unconscious, which is necessary for the patient's survival. Paintings, sculptures, or any other creative expression will reveal the crucial role the symptoms play and will allow a patient to call off the "guard dogs." Unfortunately, however, Mr. Roberts never got that far.

71

Occasionally patients with advanced cancer or some other life-threatening disease have so much trouble accepting the diagnosis and prognosis that they break with reality. When that happened at Scott & White, the oncologist, cardiologist, or other specialist who had delivered the bad news often referred the patient to Psychiatry. In fact, sometimes they were so reluctant to sit down and say, "Mr. Jones, I'm afraid you have multiple sclerosis" that they punted that responsibility to me.

Success Stories with Art Therapy

By the time a patient named Speedy Swift got to Scott & White, his cancer was so advanced that he had no more than six months to live. The adenocarcinoma (cancer that originates in the glandular tissue) had metastasized from his stomach to his liver. My colleague removed Speedy's stomach, but there was no way to stop his highly aggressive cells from doing their lethal damage elsewhere.

The day after the operation the surgeon sat down with Speedy and his wife and told them that they had not been able to get all the cells. He advised them to decide how they would like to spend the few months Speedy had left. The Swifts seemed to understand and accept the prognosis. They struck the doctor as warm and caring. At least Speedy had a loving wife and family who would give him the support and care he would need as his life came to an end. The next day the surgical resident phoned me to say that Speedy had left the hospital. His wife had found him and brought him back, but in the meantime he had purchased seven new pickup trucks. There must have been one happy salesman at a local dealership! When I told the resident that Speedy was psychotic and should be transferred to the psychiatric unit, the young physician replied, "If he were crazy, he couldn't have made such good deals on those trucks." But I prevailed, and the understanding car dealer let the family return the trucks.

From the moment Speedy walked into our unit, I could tell he was manic—totally out of control. He spoke rapidly and urgently, his face was flushed, he cracked jokes right and left, and his ideas ricocheted around the room. I laughed with him, even though I knew he was in serious trouble. To protect himself from the horrible reality of his death sentence, he had developed a full-fledged psychosis. He was out of touch with reality; if he were in touch with reality, he would have felt frightened and sad. Instead, he felt terrific. To bring him down and to allow him to sleep, I prescribed a mood-stabilizer and, at bedtime, a sedative.

When the nurse gave him his orientation to the unit, the feature that fascinated him was the creative workshop. The strong Texas sunlight streamed in through tall windows. Slogans, cartoons, and thank-you notes, all painted by the patients, covered the walls. Perched on wooden stools, patients were busily working at four by eight-foot tables with paints and big brushes scattered across them. During his ten days on the unit, Speedy spent most of his time in that workshop. He produced hundreds of paintings. The best were reminiscent of the twentieth-century French painter Braque. Speedy gave me a drawing of a horse (Below) that was so well-done that it hangs next to the fireplace in my living room not only for sentimental reasons, but also because my wife and I love it as a piece of art.

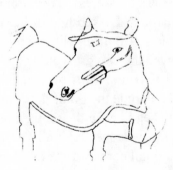

Illustration No. 2: Speedy's drawing of a horse.

Most of Speedy's subjects clearly expressed his existential dilemma of living with a disease that would soon kill him. There were abandoned cars and trucks, clocks without hands, and a wrecking ball swinging at a dilapidated apartment house. My horse had only three legs. Although Speedy could not bear to face his imminent death directly, at least he could deal with it through his art, and his emotions gave his work such strength and authenticity that we found it hard to believe that he had never painted before. He stayed in the hospital for three weeks. However, within two months Speedy Swift was dead. Although he never accepted his diagnosis, he continued painting right up until the day he died. After the funeral his wife wrote our staff and thanked them for opening up the avenue of art to him. "Without his art, he would have been out of control," she said.

Our art studio was an accessible designated space. It featured natural light, tables, and comfortable stools. When patients asked me about painting at home, I explained that setting aside a corner of a room generally does not work because chatter, visitors, television, and other distractions interfere with the creative process. I told them to find a place to paint, a place where they could make a mess. Then, all they needed was heavy paper or wall board twenty-four by thirty-six inches and thick brushes, large crayons, and big jars of acrylics. Supplies were inexpensive and readily available at art supply or hobby stores. When I entered into psychotherapy with an outpatient, I asked him or her to bring to the first session a non-realistic self-portrait and a family portrait. We then sat together and viewed the work. I would say, "Tell me about the painting." Usually I was met with resistance. "It doesn't mean anything." Rather than argue the point, I asked about some detail like the colors, a road heading for the mountains, a farmhouse that looked like a prison, a volcano beginning to erupt, or a picture that only occupied a small corner of the available space. All these were grist for the therapeutic mill.

A forty-five year-old female physician who was unable to think her way out of her second half-of-life crisis, responded well to creative therapy. Her painting (Next page) of a sailboat beached on a sand bar triggered the following dialogue:

Nancy: I have no idea what I was doing in that painting.

74

RR: What do you see?

Nancy: Well, it's a sailboat and a dock.

RR: And the sail is down.

Nancy: No one's on the boat. I must have gotten out. I felt like I was stuck there; the sailboat is grounded.

RR: Yes.

Nancy: My dad took me out in a sailboat once. He couldn't sail and he insisted on taking me out in the sailboat, but we couldn't get back. He didn't know how to get the boat back to the dock. I was getting sunburned and upset, but for hours he wouldn't give up. Why did I go out on the boat with him when I knew it wouldn't turn out right?

RR: You said before you liked to argue with him.

Nancy: So I went out in a sailboat with a man who couldn't sail just to argue? That makes no sense to me at all.

RR: It doesn't?

Nancy: Finally he climbed out of the boat—the water was only about three feet deep—and dragged the boat to shore.

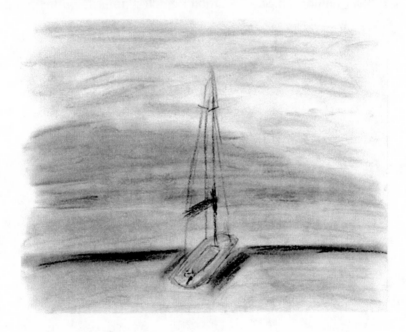

Illustration No. 3: Nancy's sailboat beached on a sandbar.

If patients brought in a lot of paintings at once, I had them select three or four to discuss. I watched carefully as they sorted through the pictures, and if I noticed a strong negative reaction to one, I made sure we included it. Many times when I asked patients to make a portrait of their current family or their family of origin, they did not include themselves. The natural follow-up was "Why did you leave yourself out?" This often opened a window into repressed emotional conflict. At other times they painted something symbolic of their family unit.

For example, let's look at John. John was a fifty-year-old surgeon who complained of depression and "burnout." He had prescribed anti-depressants for himself, but, "They cause impotence and my wife is pushing me to get psychiatric treatment." This very bright man, for whom traditional psychotherapy had failed, found insight through his paintings.

John was the oldest of four sons. At twelve he became responsible for the family because his father ran their restaurant all week and went fishing on Sunday. John depicted himself in this painting.

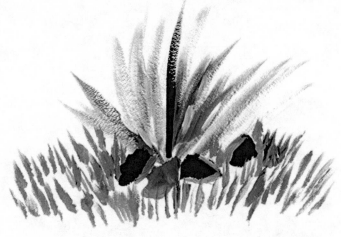

Illustration No. 4: John depicts himself in a painting.

John's artwork of rocks enabled him to see his sense of isolation and heavy responsibility and gain insight through his paintings, especially after we talked.

RR: Tell me about the painting.

76

John: Well, I don't know. It's just some rocks and some feathery things. It doesn't mean anything.

RR: Look at the rocks.

John: There are four. The one in the middle is me, I guess.

RR: You're the light-colored one?

John: Yes.

RR: And over that rock is a tall, dark column.

John: I was the one who had to hold up the family. I never got to be a kid.

RR: And that made you feel . . . ?

John: Angry—very, very angry. When I first came to this country, my parents put me in school. I didn't know the language and the only thing fit to eat was chicken. I'd never even heard of potato chips. After school I went to work in the restaurant and then home to take care of the rest of the family. Shouldn't someone have been taking care of me part of the time?

Other Art Forms as Therapy: Photographs

Personal and family photographs can reveal a lot about conflicted relationships. I realized the importance of this when I first saw a picture of my maternal grandparents on their honeymoon in 1900. The picture was taken in the hills at the Broadmoor Hotel in Colorado. My grandmother was riding sidesaddle on a donkey. She was fashionably dressed but wore a grim expression. Her new husband was holding the donkey, looking depressed in his three-piece suit and Homburg hat. Behind them was a very handsome man who was my grandfather's boss. He was the only one in the picture who looked happy. My mother could never explain why this handsome man was with her parents on their honeymoon.

My grandmother, whom we called "Ga Ga," did not want my mother to marry my father. She felt my father's family was inferior even though his father was a distinguished high school principal who was the founder of the National Honor Society. For the first time in her life, my mother defied her mother by marrying my father and leaving Pittsburgh, but Ga Ga never stopped hating him. I can't remember her ever enjoying much of anything. She was always overdressed and grim-faced, just like the photograph

77

taken on her honeymoon. If Ga Ga had come to me as a patient, I would have insisted we start her therapy by discussing this photograph as it held much information about repressed emotions.

During my medical practice one of my patients brought in a snapshot from his family vacation. The patient at about age twelve, his parents, and his six-year-old stepsister were sitting around a table in a rustic cabin. None of them was touching or looking at each other. They all stared at the camera dejectedly. Previously my patient had described his family as "very close and loving. We had great times together." Confronted with the photo, he was deeply moved by the reality depicted. They were cold, distant, unhappy people.

In another case, a young man came to see me after the birth of his first son because he was having difficulty bonding with the child. "The only feeling I have for him is irritation." He told me his father had never been close to him and that his mother had married his father because she was pregnant with his older brother and had remained in the marriage because of him and his brother. The mother complained constantly and would often declare that when the young man finished high school, she would divorce her husband. And she did. My patient felt responsible for his parents' unhappiness.

I asked him to bring old family photographs to our next session. Some weeks earlier, his mother had presented him with an album of photographs of his childhood. She suggested he make an album like this for his new son. In all of the pictures my patient looked unhappy. In several he was enraged and screaming. When I asked him about that he said, "My older brother had just bitten me." Another picture showed him as a toddler in diapers trying to pull his older brother in a wagon through deep grass. In still another he and his older brother were going out to trick or treat. His brother was dressed as a vampire, and he was a skunk. As we looked at these photos, my patient became angry. "How could my mother have chosen these pictures?" Although he had looked at them, this was the first time he had really seen them and seen the distant mother he had grown up with.

I was struck by a photo from his college graduation. My

gowned patient stood with his divorced mother and father. For the first time, his mother was smiling and was clearly happy, as was his father. My patient was not. He also brought photographs of his current family. In one he and his attractive wife were holding their son. They were smiling. I asked my patient to describe his expression. "My expression is that I can't accept that I'm a father," he said. "My body language says I want to be out of the picture." Building on these insights, we spent our remaining sessions addressing the young man's main goal which was to stop the pattern of parental rejection in which he was trapped. I had him paint family portraits and pictures of his dreams. As we worked together, he became able to enjoy playing with his little boy, even to feel comfortable changing his son's diaper, and he continued to paint.

Poetry as Therapy

Requiring nothing more than a pencil and a sheet of paper, poetry can provide another rapid route to repressed emotions. Some people write poems routinely, others only during periods of joy or stress. I always asked patients if they had ever written poems. If they said yes, I encouraged them to share their poems with me. The following is an example of poetry as therapy.

Diana had a rare psychiatric condition which was then called multiple personality disorder; she had two separate personalities. The goal we agreed upon was for the two personalities to become one. We ultimately achieved that goal with hypnosis, which I will come back to later. I received a poem Diana wrote several months into her therapy. Here is an excerpt:

Skin Hunger

I read today that the SKIN is the largest ORGAN in the body—skin is an organ system. Other organs have needs/requirements in order to be healthy. The heart needs blood.

The lungs need air.

The stomach needs food

The brain needs stimulation through sight, sound, and thought.

The muscles need exercise

Skin needs touch.

What happens when one is deprived of touching, hugging–stroking? Newborns, according to Reneé Spitz, who do not receive adequate touching, loving, nurturing may die—even if fed and sheltered. Psychology students learn about the study by Harlow, who took monkeys away from their natural mothers and gave them cloth or wire substitutes with feeding nipples–but none of the mother's fur, heartbeat, or movement–and the monkeys developed serious problems—physical malaise and socially maladjusted skills—some died. If a newborn needs touching, does an adult, do I?

I can rarely recall being touched in a gentle, nurturing manner–touch meant pain. Childhood memories do not include hugs, kisses, cuddling. They are shrouded in secrets, perverse sexual acts, crude hands—

there were no whisper touches

and now my skin screams

Please touch me

Don't touch me

Please don't hurt me

A physician would diagnose my condition as "skin hunger." I suffer from

"stroke deprivation." I have never been touched lovingly, nurturingly—never enough.

I am hungry.

I wonder how different I would be if I had been touched, held, stroked—loved just a little?

But I will be

Always fleeing,

Always waiting.

When shall I confront my fears, my images, images—secretly related.

Creating

Or

Destroying

in life

in dreams

in art

or

by touch? Alone!

This poem helped both Diana and me understand her fear of abandonment and lead us more quickly into insight and transcendence. Another patient, Betsy, an intelligent mentally ill woman, drove twelve hundred miles round-trip for our weekly appoint-

ments. She believed her poetry had helped save her the way
Jung's creative activities had saved him from a psychosis. Here is
an excerpt from one of her poems:

I walked up a long
flight
of stairs, today.
As I waited for an
answer
at the door, I thought
"This is your chance,
JUMP!"
I looked down—
calculated that it was not high enough—yet.
My imagination
ran away with
me—it was almost
exhilarating—in a
terrifying way.
Then from some
rational
part of me—
a message
NO
Something—a force
pushed me toward the
door
away
from the railing
as the door was opening.

This patient obviously was grappling with suicidal impulses,
and her poem expressed the reassurance she felt on experiencing the counterbalancing, rational side of herself holding her back
from self-destruction. As Betsy dealt with her repressed conflicts
and became more integrated, we negotiated the termination of
therapy. Not surprisingly, she felt ambivalent about this. She was
gratified by her progress, happy to be relieved of her depression,
but also fearful of separating from me. When we discussed her
poems, Betsy recognized that she had never been allowed to be
dependent. Even as a little girl, she had been pushed to achieve in

school, to fulfill the expectations of others. Thanks to the insight she had gained through therapy, she was able to re-experience the denial of her dependency needs and recognize and even celebrate them. She could join the child she had never been allowed to be, in the patch of bright, fresh clover she had created for herself in a poem she sent to me after her sessions ended.

Hypnotism

Another tool for successful therapy was hypnosis. The potential for hypnotism has intrigued European and American doctors since the late eighteenth century when Viennese physician Franz Anton Mesmer refined the technique in a celebrated but unsuccessful attempt to demonstrate what he called animal magnetism. Because the blood contained iron, he posited that cures of various ailments could be achieved through the use of magnets to correct imbalances. An essential part of this treatment involved Dr. Mesmer sitting close to patients, looking deep into their eyes, and asking them to concentrate on shiny objects which he swung or rotated slowly as he announced that the patient's complaints would vanish when they woke up. Many of his patients made remarkable recoveries, but it was his hypnotic technique of "mesmerism," not the magnets, that affected the cures.

Half a century later, American healer P. P. Quimby learned mesmerism and used it to cure Mary Baker Eddy's hysterical paralysis, allowing Christian Science to be born. French physician Jean-Martin Charcot cured hysterical conversion disorders with this hypnotic technique, helping his student Sigmund Freud to understand the psychodynamics of denial and repression. Although hysteria is more likely to show up today as back pain than as the pseudo-seizures common in Freud's day, hypnosis remains a powerful therapeutic tool to help cure the conversion symptoms caused by inner conflicts.

Generally speaking, removing conflict-producing symptoms is possible when the symptoms are no longer needed to protect the patient from the conflict. Suggested removal of some noxious symptom such as pain was almost always successful. More complicated issues like addiction to food, tobacco or alcohol were usually resistant to treatment by hypnosis because those addictions required the patient to take a risk. If the patient was not motivated, he or she would not accept the hypnotic suggestion.

But the removal of pain by hypnosis is dramatic. I hypnotized Marjie when she delivered our third son: She went to sleep during the contractions and woke up when they subsided. She experienced no pain, and her blood pressure, pulse, and respirations were normal. In that situation she was eager to accept the suggestions.

In the course of my practice, I found hypnosis effective with a broad range of patients, including those with previously mentioned multiple personality disorder—one of the rarest and most complex diagnoses. At forty-two, my patient Diana, author of the poem "Skin Hunger," had no memory of her childhood that several family members told me had been marked by severe verbal, physical, and sexual abuse. Her alter personality, Donna, had endured this abuse and would take over when Diana waas threatened. She became Donna the Protector. But Dianna wanted her childhood memories, and she wanted to integrate Donna. "She embarrasses me when she's out," Diana explained.

I suggested videotaping a hypnotic session and she agreed. When Diana was in a trance, I asked her to allow Donna to come out. When Donna came out she was angry and defensive. Her voice, demeanor, and attitude were totally unlike Diana's. Not surprisingly, Donna was quite hostile because my involvement was a threat to her very existence. When I related Diana's goal in order to find her past, Donna contemptuously reported that the last time Diana had been hospitalized in our unit Donna had taken over and made things so difficult for her doctor that he dismissed her as a patient. In fact, he dismissed her from the unit entirely. I told Donna that was when my colleague asked me to take over Diana's care. Then I said to Donna, "Now we're going to hypnotize you and allow Diana to come back." She reluctantly agreed and finally accepted my suggestion. When I brought her out of the trance, she was Diana, but she had no conscious awareness of

Donna telling her of her past.

It wasn't until Diana viewed the video tape that she became frightened and fascinated by her memories. Through a series of hypnotic sessions, we eventually achieved the goal of transcendence, moving past her emotional, repressed memories. Diana and Donna united. Whenever she needed to get in touch with those repressed experiences, she viewed the tapes.

Hypnosis was effective in the case of another patient, Martha, as well. She was a moderately obese young woman the police brought into the emergency room. She appeared dazed and disheveled. The emergency room physician who had examined her told me she had been charged with abandoning a newborn baby at the altar of the First Methodist Church. A concerned janitor reported her to the police. She told the police that she had never been pregnant and was certain there was some terrible mistake. Her physical exam showed that she had recently delivered a child. She was then admitted to the psychiatric unit.

As I looked into Martha's background, I discovered that she lived alone and worked as an aide in a local nursing home. Her employer described her as a quiet, hard worker and did not believe she had been pregnant. Martha was frightened by her involvement with the law and agreed to a videotaped hypnotic session "if it will settle things with the police." While hypnotized she gave a complete account of her pregnancy. The father was a soldier who had been transferred to Louisiana shortly after their brief liaison. Martha recounted wearing baggy clothing to hide her pregnancy and then delivering the baby in her bathtub after arranging toweling, clamps, and scissors. Labor and delivery took about three hours. She then disposed of the placenta, which the police found later in the garbage. Wrapping the baby in a blanket without even checking to see whether it was a boy or a girl, she took it to the church. During the entire session Martha expressed no emotion. When she awakened she did not want to see the tape but did accept our report that she had delivered a baby and agreed to put it up for adoption. "I want to go back to work, when all this legal stuff is over," she declared. The powerful psychological defense of repression and isolation had protected her from any feelings.

84

She was immune to any grief about the loss of the child. When she was dismissed she asked me this question: "If I actually had that baby, why didn't my milk come down?"

Most children are wonderful hypnotic subjects because an important thing about hypnosis is that there can be no question about the fact of its effectiveness. One evening I was in the emergency room admitting a psychotic patient to our psychiatric unit when I heard a terrified child screaming. Curious, I looked into the room and saw my orthopedic surgeon friend Dr. Sandy Lowry trying to help a nine-year-old boy with a fractured leg. The boy, Conrad, was still in his soccer uniform. He was terrified. His father, a cardiologist of my acquaintance, was extremely upset. I asked him if I could help and told him I would be willing to hypnotize his son so Sandy could reduce the fracture and apply the cast. Both he and Dr. Lowry thought this was a great idea. So, after taking off my white coat and my tie because Conrad was so frightened of the doctors who were not able to manage him, I sat down next to him and told him I was there to help him.

When I said that I was going to hypnotize him, Conrad stopped screaming and said, "Can you really hypnotize me?"

"Sure," I replied. "Nothing to it. Here's what we do. Tell me your favorite place."

"The beach."

"Now, close your eyes and imagine that you're on the beach. You can feel the hot sun and hear the waves and feel the warm sand." Once I could see that Conrad had transported himself, in his imagination, to the beach, I began a series of suggestions:

"You are very, very sleepy. You can't keep your eyes open. As you get sleepy you take three deep breaths, and with each breath you go into a deeper sleep. Now that you've taken these deep breaths, you find you are on the top of an elevator that goes down ten floors and with each floor you go down, you become deeper and deeper asleep. So you're on the ninth floor, feeling sleepy, then the eighth floor as you become deeper asleep. When you get to the basement, you are sound asleep and relaxed. And now that you are deeply asleep and completely relaxed, you're going to feel your left leg completely relaxed. It will feel weightless and will float up off the table. Dr. Lowry will fix your leg and put a cast on it, but you won't feel any of that."

Like most kids, he had accepted these suggestions and soon was in a profound trance, following my every suggestion. His leg remained elevated for the entire procedure. When Dr. Lowry was finished, I told Conrad that on the count of three he would be wide awake. Upon awakening he said, "When my friends sign my cast, I can tell them about being hypnotized!" As a result of the success of this hypnosis, Dr. Lowry and I talked about my teaching hypnosis to his department and his residents.

During my residency at Mayo, my psychiatrist friend and teacher Dr. Ed Litin and I tried hypnosis in a much more serious situation. We were seeing a young woman who had been admitted with a conversion symptom called hysterical aphonia. She was unable to speak, or even to whisper. She communicated by writing notes. After we obtained an incomplete psychiatric history, Dr. Litin told her that if, and only if she no longer needed the symptom to preserve her psychological equilibrium, he could remove it with hypnosis. He reassured her that it would be okay to keep the aphonia if she thought it was necessary to preserve her emotional integrity. She shook her head vigorously and hurriedly wrote, "Please hypnotize me!"

As soon as Dr. Litin began the hypnosis, the patient went under. As she did, tears began streaming down her face. Ed looked at me, pointed to the tears, and brought the woman out of the trance. In response to her disappointment, he explained that the tears meant that she still required the emotional protection the symptom provided and that we needed more time to explore her inner conflict before removing her symptom. Ed Litin, always an incredible teacher, said, "Never raise more dust than you can settle!" In avoiding raising that unmanageable dust he stressed the importance of physiologic clues, like a blush, the rising pitch of a patient's voice, a deep sigh. "And until you've spent time with a patient," he cautioned, "you should respect the potential for loss of control." We did not know enough about the patient's problems to rush into uncovering unconscious material.

Chapter Seven
Connecting with the Unconscious

Yet another way for me to explore what patients were going through was by evaluating and discussing their dreams with them. The fact is that all of us connect with our unconscious through our dreams. The characters, situations, objects, even the colors that appear in our dreams are all expressions of important messages from our unconscious. Having my patient describe a dream, including the feelings provoked in and by it, was an extremely valuable tool for me to help my patients obtain insight.

Benjamin Rush, father of American psychiatry and one of the signers of the Declaration of Independence, listened to his own inner voices as closely as he did to those of his patients. In 1785 during a time of national triumph, he dreamed that a great crowd was surging about Christ Church in Philadelphia, and he approached the group. A man had climbed the steeple and was sitting on the ball just below the weather vane. Rush asked what was happening, and he was told that the man on the steeple had discovered he could control the weather. He could call up the sun and rain and cause the wind to blow from any direction. In effect, he claimed mastery of the weather vane. It was no longer an indicator; it was a direction instrument. The man held a trident in his hand like Neptune and flourished it as he shouted his commands.

Alas, the elements refused to comply. He called for the rain; the sun shone, and the streets were dry. He called for the wind; Philadelphia was becalmed. The trident wielder, after a while, showed signs of agitation, and then he sank into a deep depression. "The man is extremely mad," the doctor told a friend in the dream. At this moment a messenger dressed like Mercury descended from the steeple carrying a banner. Dr. Rush read the Latin device, *De te fibula narrator*, which translates to "About you a story is being told."

Rush wrote in his account of the dream: "The impression of these words was so forcible on my mind that I instantly awoke, and from that time I determined never to attempt to influence the opinions and passions of my fellow citizens upon political subjects." In his prompt reading of the dream Rush recognized both within sleep and on his awakening who the trident wielder on the steeple was. It was himself.

People often claim that they never dream. Many believe that when they are asleep, their brain is turned off, but the unconscious is always active. In a sleep study laboratory subjects were awakened when they entered the dreaming state or REM (rapid eye movements). They then related the dreams into a tape recorder. In the morning they typically reported that they had no dreams, but the tape had recorded seven or eight different dreams.

Throughout recorded history dreams have been important in understanding unconscious inner conflicts. Not surprisingly, dreams claim major spots in the traditions and myths of the world's cultures. The Hebrew scriptures tell of Joseph being released from prison and then, virtually overnight, becoming the second most powerful man in Egypt because he correctly interpreted the pharaoh's prophetic dream of seven years of plenty and seven years of drought. Further, dreams were associated with healing in the ancient Greek healing centers such as the Temple of Asclepius, named for the god of healing. Physicians in these healing centers asked patients about their dreams and interpreted a serpent appearing in a dream as a sign that healing had begun. Down to the present, the physicians' sign is a serpent ascending a staff.

On numerous occasions, patients have told me their prophetic dreams. One such example is a woman who was troubled by a dream she had before her breast biopsy. She saw herself on the shore of a vast ocean trying to tell her husband that he could not go with her on her journey. He would not listen to her even though she begged him to pay attention. When she told him the dream, he dismissed it, but I did not. Together, my patient and I explored the dream's symbolism of death and loss. In less than a year she died of breast cancer, but she and I had been able to deal with the feelings her dream had made accessible. She benefitted by reading Ernest Becker's book, *The Denial of Death*, which proved to be an excellent facilitator for our discussions. On our last visit she talked about her prophetic dream. "The most tragic aspect," she said, "was that it accurately foretold that I would not be able to say goodbye to my husband."

At age fifteen my fourth son related two dreams to us at breakfast one morning. In the first he said he was frantically looking through his wallet for his ID cards. "I could find my older brother's but not mine," he said. In his other dream he and some of his friends went to a train station to take a trip. He knew that before he could continue his journey, he had to kill the old lady who lived in a little shack down by the tracks. At this point Marjie said, "It's okay. Just go. You don't have to kill me." We all laughed but she realized he had to separate from her and wanted to make it clear she wasn't going to try to stop him.

In *The Body Has a Head* Gustav Eckstein writes about a dream recounted by physiologist Dr. Otto Loewi, the discoverer of one of the neurotransmitters. In 1904, Loewi had read a paper describing an experiment by a scientist named Weber who had stopped a frog's heart by stimulating the vagus nerve. Loewi had been struggling for seventeen years to figure out the biochemical mechanism by which that could have happened. Then, two nights before Easter Sunday, he awoke from a dream. While he was still groggy he wrote down a description on a scrap of paper in hopes of figuring it out the following morning. When he read his note the next day, it made no sense, but that night he awoke at three a.m. with two clear recollections—one of his recent dream, the other of the paper he had read in 1904. In Eckstein's book he writes, "The dream was a completed experiment. It was instructions printed in Loewi's mind as in a laboratory manual. He got up. He went to the laboratory and performed the experiment on the hearts of two frogs." For seventeen years Lowei's mind had struggled to solve this problem until finally his unconscious revealed the answers through his dream.

Dream Interpretation of Carl Jung

Carl Jung and Sigmund Freud differed in their approaches to the interpretation of dreams. Freud was always the authority. He

91

decided what the dream meant and developed his own symbolic imagery. Jung, on the other hand, gave the patient the authority for interpretation. The dream meant what it meant to the dreamer.

In my dream work I followed Jung's approach. When my patients had dreams, I asked them to record them upon awakening and then to paint them. A young woman, Samantha, came to see me because her husband had left her and their three children saying he did not love her any more. She painted a dream in which she was looking down on their living room. Her husband was curled up in the fetal position on the floor in front of the TV. Their three little girls were playing in another part of the room (Illustration No. 5). When I asked her what the dream meant, she replied that her husband was unable to participate in the family because he was incapable of intimate relationships, not because, as she had believed before, that there was something flawed in her. That was a significant insight. By following Jung's approach to dreams, I insisted Samantha tell me what she saw instead of my telling her what the symbols represented.

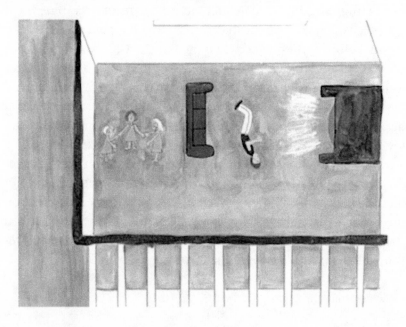

Illustration No. 5: Samantha's living room.

Two weeks later Samantha dreamed that she accompanied her husband to a swimming pool. He excitedly told her he had devised a way to re-breathe his own oxygen under water and wanted her to time how long he could stay submerged. After an incredibly long time, he surfaced and asked how long he had been under. Then he asked her to time him again. When he resurfaced, she told him the second submersion was one second longer than the first. The husband insisted on continuing this activity to improve his time, but Samantha refused because she remembered the children were with a new babysitter, and she needed to get back to them.

Samantha painted the dream as a portrait of her husband under water, his eyes closed, his earplugs in place, and a blissful expression on his face. She told me he had become obsessive about exercise and devoted all his time to running, so much so that she was very concerned about his health. "He's running all the time," she said. She felt the need to confront him with his obvious self-destructiveness. "If he were as obsessed with drugs or alcohol, I would try to commit him," she said.

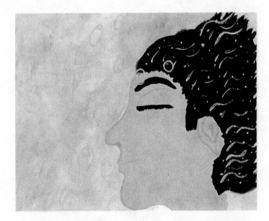

Illustration No. 6:
Samantha's husband,
under water.

Samantha arranged a meeting for the three of us. When her husband viewed the painting, he agreed that he was totally isolating himself from the world and recognized that he was self-destructive. As he looked at his wife's portrait of him, he said with tears filling his voice, "I need to be in a hospital." His wife and I supported him in this, and I told him I would make arrangements for psychiatric care for him.

Carl Jung thought that dreams had an important compensatory effect. If a person consciously believed she was superior in every way, her dream might be of sewage backing up and filling the bathtub. Conversely, self-deprecating patients with low self-esteem often had healing dreams in which they received awards. In addition to hastening insight, then, dreams can help balance the inner self.

Having patients draw and relate their dreams proved to be one of my most productive psychotherapeutic tools. Like art, dreams are the product of the patients' unconscious, so they cannot resist the dream's implications as something external or imposed. An example of this situation is Janet, a successful businesswoman in her sixties, who came to me for help with her depression and her conflicted relationship with her grown son. I gave her an assignment: "Keep a sketch pad and pencil by your bed. If you wake from a dream in the middle of the night, or recall a dream when you wake up in the morning, draw it immediately."

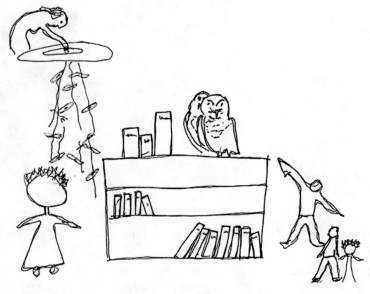

Illustration No. 7: Janet's owl drawing.

One day Janet brought in a sketch. (Previous page) It had several people in it and two owls, one partly hidden behind the other. What follows is our conversation about the drawing and the dream, given in complete form here simply to show how listening and guiding can take people where they would never go on their own while at the same time reaching the mutual goal of obtaining insight.

RR: Tell me about your dream.

Janet: I went on a house call with my son to help him sell something. The customer was strange, didn't say much. The customer asked my son if he could accept the briefcase he'd promised to give him. My son said 'yes.' The man said he'd order it. Then a hole opened up in the ceiling, and the man's wife threw down paper plates, cups, and tableware. The man then reached toward a white owl that was sitting on top of the bookcase. When the owl moved, I could see there was a second owl right behind him. My mother sat quietly on one side of the room. My son and the man and I were on another. The man's wife tried to get through the door, but she was too large. I stepped aside to let her through.

RR: You and your son were making the house call. What do you associate with that?

Janet: Well, I help him with his business sometimes.

RR: Was this person on the house call likely to buy from you?

Janet: He was rich. He was giving my son an expensive briefcase.

RR: But was he interested in buying?

Janet: We never talked about that, so probably not.

RR: You said he was strange. Tell me more about that.

Janet: He was very cool towards me—wouldn't look at me, wouldn't answer my questions about what kind of work he did.

RR: Did you recognize him?

Janet: No.

RR: Then the rule of thumb is he probably represented a part of you.

Janet: He was a little feminine.

RR: And strange. He wouldn't look at you or talk to you. What about that?

Janet: He was closing me out. I don't know why.

RR: You were in an awkward position. You were trying to help your son and this rich man was trying to give him a briefcase. What was your role?

Janet: The briefcase was their business. I wasn't in on it. He wasn't giving me a briefcase.

RR: You were left out.

Janet: I wasn't upset about it in the dream. But I did notice my mother was sitting across the room, not saying anything. She was left out, too, I guess.

RR: Do you have any associations with your mother and a rich man?

Janet: I don't think this was about my mother and the man. I felt like she was watching me more than becoming involved in the meeting.

RR: You're not answering my question.

Janet: Because I don't want to go there.

RR: You'd better go there.

Janet: We had family friends—my mother had family friends—the guy was rich and he was also a pervert. But I don't see what that has to do with my son's business.

RR: Are you sure your dream is about your son's business?

Janet: No.

RR: What do you think it really was about?

Janet: Maybe my mother always telling me what to do, always getting in the way of me not doing what I wanted to do.

RR: And this man is married. Tell me about his wife.

Janet: She was a big woman, couldn't have children, adopted a little girl, went to the movies all the time, and she hired my older sister to help her clean her house on Saturday mornings. Never hired me. She was not a warm, loving person by a long shot. I remember being shamed by her when I waved at some guys in a train. She also made me a beautiful dress one time, the only thing she had ever sewn.

RR: And she was throwing things at you through a hole in the ceiling?

Janet: Just the tableware. She brought the food through the door later in the dream.

RR: What do you associate with that?

Janet: They had Sunday dinner with us every Sunday when I was growing up. Her husband also gave my dad a lot of stuff. She gave my mother stuff, too. She was always redecorating her house and giving us the old stuff.

RR: You had the feeling she was above you.

Janet: Always, and in the dream too.

RR: You had to step aside to let her into the room.

Janet: She was fat. I hated her.

RR: Can you put this together?

Janet: I think the two owls are saying something to me. Maybe there is wisdom hiding back behind what I always thought was true.

RR: And there are two owls. The man moves the first one, and there's another one behind it. What do you associate with that?

96

Janet: I didn't see the second one at first. I thought there was only one, the one that was his, the one he wanted to come sit on his shoulder. But there was another one.

RR: Let's look at the drawing. Tell me what you see.

Janet: The guy's wife throwing stuff down from a hole in the ceiling. My mother is below her. The guy is reaching for the owl, but he's tiny and can't reach the top of the bookcase. My son and I are watching him, actually we're not watching him.

RR: No, you're not. Comment about the size differential.

Janet: I thought the most important thing in the dream was the owl sitting on a case full of books.

RR: Are there names on the books?

Janet: No, I was just trying to do a good drawing and make them look like real books.

RR: What do you associate with books?

Janet: That I haven't read enough.

RR: There are a lot of empty spaces in the bookshelf.

Janet: Those are the ones I haven't read.

RR: How are you going to achieve wisdom?

Janet: I don't know. I guess I feel wise in a lot of ways but . . .

RR: But you still can't leave your mother and the strange neighbor.

Janet: At my advanced age I still find myself saying, "Well, maybe this will please my mother." That's sick. I'd also feel a lot better if I could grab the man's privates and twirl him around until they fell off.

RR: You have a lot of anger.

Janet: If I'd been smarter, I never would have let that happen.

RR: Your mother didn't protect you?

Janet: No. I told her about him, but she didn't believe me. He was inappropriate with my younger sister as well, but I didn't know that until we were all grown up.

RR: Do you think it was wise to take your son to that house? What was the message?

Janet: Was I leading him down the wrong path by helping him with his business? Shouldn't I have left him alone to do his own thing? This man we were visiting was a pervert. But I didn't let him go alone.

RR: You said you weren't smart enough not to go there, but maybe in going back there you and your son will find some wisdom.

Janet: We'll each have our own pet owl?

RR: Yes.

Rather than undergoing years of psychoanalysis to uncover the trauma of that early sexual abuse and her subsequent feelings of helplessness, abandonment, and self-blame, Janet had reached the breakthrough to those long-repressed experiences and emotions in just a few sessions. It does not always happen quite that fast, but often it does. Her long-repressed feelings were traumatic, and she had constructed her life around avoiding them, but because Janet's own dreams had revealed them, and her own drawing had depicted them, her resistance was minimal. I was able to guide her past it with a few gentle questions. At our next session, Janet reported feeling markedly better. She felt affirmed, rather than stupid. She made an effort not to obsess about little things. She had several warm interactions with each of her children, and she was optimistic about her future. The energy that her unconscious mind had consumed in the effort to keep those repressed emotions locked up was now available to her for living. I spent the subsequent two sessions helping her access her grief for her mother that had been blocked by Janet's locked-down anger at her betrayal.

I have always trusted my own dreams to give me direction even though I do not always like the message. After our nest emptied we rented a place in Chicago so Marjie could pursue her acting and writing career. When we realized after about ten years that we needed more room than her tiny rental, we started looking for a larger downtown loft. As we looked, I was smitten by a large space over a bookstore which was far above our budget. Marjie didn't want to buy it partly because of the cost, but also because she thought it much too large, a bit scary, and she didn't like the layout of the rooms. I, however, had the bit in my teeth. I explained to the owner that I was going to be out in the wilderness canoeing with my sons and would not be able to communicate with him until I returned. I said to him, "If you can sell it before I come back, fine, but we will make you an offer when I return in two weeks."

On the third night of our trip, I had a powerful dream. In the dream I was in an extremely long Cadillac convertible, and I knew that everyone would admire me in this beautiful car. I soon realized I could not easily steer the car, and the brakes didn't work at all. Then it began to rain, turning into a downpour but, despite my frantic attempts, I could not raise the roof of the convertible. The next morning I told my son Jim about the dream and he said,

"Dad, your dream seems to be telling you not to buy that loft." I nodded yes. "But I'm still going to buy it."

Jim said, "Dad, is that wise?" Experiencing some anger as my bite loosened from my bit, separating myself from this wonderful loft, I replied, "No, it isn't wise." We did not buy the loft.

Existential Shock Therapy

For years, I recommended Irvin Yalom's textbook *Existential Psychotherapy* published by Basic Books to my residents and patients. It includes a number of illuminating exercises including one he calls existential shock therapy. Designed to jar a patient into existential awareness, it begins with the patient drafting his or her own obituary. The patient draws a straight line with birth at one end and death at the other and marks with a cross where he or she is at the present moment on that continuum. This forces the patient to focus on the time remaining, which is a powerful incentive to overcome denial, and participate actively in therapy. It is also an incentive to avoid wasting the precious years he or she has left.

I also liked to conduct another of Yalom's existential shock therapy exercises, one that was very useful even for people not experiencing particular emotional distress because it helped clarify personal priorities. I instructed the participants to tear a sheet of white paper into eight roughly equal pieces, and to write on each piece the roles with which he or she most deeply identified such as mother, golfer, friend, teacher. I then told the person taking the test to put the eight definitions in order, with the most important characteristic on the bottom. One of my especially self-aware patients found his most important role was "drinker." He listed nothing that implied relationships with others. He was a loner.

In another case, I asked a women to list her roles, and they all involved relationships with other people. Her chart looked like the one on page one hundred.

After she had put the chart together, I presented a hypothetical situation to her: "Suppose the doctor tells you that your laboratory values show that you have a lethal and untreatable condition, and

99

you have only three months to live. Now, turn over the top piece of paper. Imagine that you have to give up that role, that part of yourself, and let all your feelings come to the surface. You'll have thirty seconds to ponder each loss."

When she was finished with that, I said, "The doctor called and said that it was all a mistake. He apologized profusely, and says to tell you you're fine."

MOTHER	ARTIST
WIFE	VOLUNTEER
SISTER	ACTRESS
MENTOR	GRANDMOTHER

With this reprieve, I asked her to go through the pile again, beginning at the bottom, and again to allow all her feelings to surface but this time she should be open to her feelings about the roles she had regained. Almost invariably, test-takers such as this patient stopped after reclaiming the bottom three or four because they realized that was all that was really important. They recognized the remaining four or five as accessories and could then focus on the most important issues relating to their goals for psychotherapy.

Periodically I conduct the test on myself. Yalom's exercises are especially helpful with physician patients. Among doctors, the most common psychological complaint is existential burn-out. Running a close second is drug and alcohol dependence. Sometimes they are combined. During my time as chairman of the Department of Psychiatry at Scott & White Clinic, doctors frequently came to me with their emotional problems. Sometimes their wives or grown children would pressure them to seek help. Sometimes the doctors themselves recognized that their growing dependence on alcohol or drugs could threaten their careers. They knew that whatever their problems, I would not be judgmental.

I have often wondered why every physician doesn't seek psychotherapy routinely. Most of us suffer from some degree of grandiosity. We think we can help people, even find a cure for a disease that has troubled mankind for millennia. The respect accorded to us by patients and the general community feeds our narcissism and our sense of omnipotence. Nowadays, the average lawyer and the well-established plumbing contractor may make much more than physicians do, but mothers still dream of their sons and daughters becoming doctors. So when a physician experiences frustrations and disappointments, the fall from the pedestal can be especially hard. When the sense of mission deserts us, when our professional belief system is rattled, we need help as much as, and maybe more, than those in another occupation.

When I scheduled a physician for psychotherapy, I explained in our first interview that it was crucial that our relationship strive toward the expression of feelings rather than a display of competency and intellectual one-upmanship. "If we play chess, you are going to win," I would say. Almost invariably this brought a tight smile. "So do you want to win, or do you want help?" I asked.

One of my surgeon friends came to me complaining of "feeling lost." He was widely respected among his colleagues and was genuinely interested in his patients as people. Born and reared in Australia and married to a Canadian woman, he told me he and his wife had "always felt like alien corn in Texas." When he took the Yalom existential exercise he was profoundly moved. The characteristic he gave the most important position was "composer," not "surgeon" or "father." As a young man, he had played the piano but put that aside when he went to medical school. He remembered his father, a general practitioner, who had his office in his home and would not allow George to play the piano for fear of bothering his patients. Both George's parents had been demanding and unaffectionate.

After completing the Yalom exercise, he resumed playing the piano and composing music. In a year he retired from surgery. Although he was still in his late fifties, his children were grown so he no longer had to worry about paying for their educations. He and his wife moved to Ireland where she opened a teashop and he composed music. He still sends me tapes of his latest compositions. The music is modern, atonal, and highly creative, not the sort of tightly structured, conventional work one would expect from a retired surgeon.

Chapter Eight
Healing by Listening

Listening to Myself

Although each patient is unique, the process of getting to a point where I could suggest what I call the "superhighway to insight" was similar for all of them. To gain insight, an individual had to be willing to go where he or she had to go for healing. He or she had to be willing to take risks. And I had to be willing to listen, really listen, not just be present during the sessions.

Every detail about a patient provides valuable insights into his or her personality. For example, sometimes the patient's occupation reveals cues. Lawyers and judges are likely to have grown up in families marked by favoritism and injustice. Many veterinarians, especially some female vets, are rejected by their parents and can trust only animals. Often physicians, when they were children of ten or eleven, had a beloved grandparent die or a sibling suffer serious injury. Some nurses did not receive enough nurturing as children. Perhaps their mothers were nurses and did not give them enough care. Policemen are often struggling with their own anti-social impulses. The stereotype of the psychiatrist or clinical psychologist as constantly grappling with his or her emotional dysfunction is painfully apt.

I noticed everything I could about a new patient, and I also kept myself acutely aware of my own feelings. I listened to myself. This provided me with important information. Doctors and other therapists often hesitate to admit their feelings, especially negative ones. From our student days on we are told, "You shouldn't get angry at a patient. It's unprofessional. Keep your own feelings out of it." But, of course, the moment I met someone I had feelings about that person, one way or another.

I often reacted because there was something in the patient that reminded me of a characteristic I did not like in myself. If my patient provoked an immediate reaction of anger, it was probably for one of three reasons: the patient was narcissistic, dependent, or sociopathic. Those are the three characteristics that most of us have never dealt with in ourselves, and we become angry when we see them in someone who is not troubled by their presence.

Narcissistic people are totally involved with their own self-love. They are consumed with their own opinion of themselves. One day at my health club, I overheard a sweaty-chested muscle man discussing the inconvenience he had the night before with his girlfriend. He said to his equally sweaty friend that he had kicked his girl out. He told her when they started to date that she could stay as long as she made him happy, but she was not making him happy anymore, so she had to go. His friend thought that was totally reasonable behavior. The girlfriend meanwhile was sobbing so hard in the next room that she was unable to lead our aerobics class.

In medical school, whenever I took a break from my studies, my very dependent roommate would ask me to get him a glass of milk or make him a peanut butter and jelly sandwich. I would quietly get furious because he was so obvious about his need to be dependent and, of course, I had some dependency issues of my own. I wanted him to do the same thing for me, but could never ask for it.

Sociopaths also are only interested in themselves, but unlike the narcissistic person, they are often involved in criminal activities. One of our son's best childhood friends broke into our neighbor's house and stole a TV set, then went to our son's apartment and stole a "not-yet-out-of-the-box" DVD player to plug into it. When the friend was found out, he blamed our son. I became very angry at him because he was a sociopath who did not experience guilt. If I felt happy when first meeting a patient, chances were excellent that the person was manic. If I had no particular feeling about a patient, he or she was probably paranoid.

I stood six feet and seven inches tall, and my size tended to reassure patients that I was in control. However, on a few occasions, I was the one who felt frightened when I first met a patient. When my first reaction to a patient was fear, I knew that I was facing an individual who was capable of violence and under, at best, marginal control. At some level I knew I was concerned about

104

my own self-control. Furthermore, being present when someone loses emotional control can be frightening. That may actually be how we are hardwired; it's a way to protect ourselves from attack, but I suspect it is also a matter of culture. We Americans imported the famous British stiff upper lip and the Northern European stoicism. Whatever the case, I learned to listen to my own emotions in providing information to treat patients

Staff members on psychiatric units learn quickly how to manage violent and potentially violent patients or they soon request a transfer. I learned that patients who lost control had no fear of doing so. Their reality was internal. Their psychosis dominated their world, and it served as a refuge. To an outside observer they might appear calm, while the voices they heard in their heads were urging them to take irrational action that could be self-destructive or hurtful to others. So, the foremost rule in a psychiatric setting was to create a safe, secure environment for distressed patients. If a patient feared loss of control, my staff and I would reassure them that nothing terrible would happen if they did so. They would simply be expressing normal emotions.

For inpatients that meant inviting the patient into a seclusion room and telling him or her to "lose control, go crazy!" The room was next to a nurses' station and featured a big window and padded walls and floor. Pillows and other soft objects were strewn about. Although the room was soundproof, a video camera and a window allowed the staff to see what was going on. For outpatients, I often recommended that they drive into the country, find a nice place to park by the side of the road, and then let go—scream, pound the steering wheel, beat fists against the seat. In both settings the loss of control resembled a temper tantrum of a three-year-old. Afterwards, they felt relief; they did not go crazy. Watching my own reactions to all different patients and situations helped me to read and understand patients and begin guided therapy.

When a patient was sent to me by a fellow physician, I would read the chart and notes that accompanied the referral. They might have told me about underlying chronic conditions or acute prob-

105

lems such as injuries, but mainly the charts warned me that the patient might be upset at being referred to a psychiatrist. He might have had a cardiac arrhythmia or an acute abdominal pain. When the cardiologist or the gastroenterologist could not find the cause, a referral to a psychiatrist could be interpreted as dismissive, as an accusation that there was nothing really wrong, that the problem was "all in your head." In cases like these, I knew I had to assure the patient right from the start that I took his or her problem seriously. My goal was to encourage patients to open up and talk, and to offer them the therapy of compassionate listening.

Beginning a Dialogue with Patients

There is no such thing as a typical or routine patient. But I did conduct sessions in an orderly and established way that suited my purposes and those of my patients. During a first session with a patient, I began by asking, "How can I help?" Sometimes, especially with female patients, that was all they needed. No one had ever invited them to tell their story, and once I did, the floodgates opened. Within forty-five minutes they gave me their complete story of trying unsuccessfully to please a distant father or a controlling mother or being made to feel guilty, even evil, because their emotionally damaged parents were not able to appreciate them or make them feel secure. If their story slowed down, I would ask them to tell me about their parents, their grandparents, and their great-grandparents. Emotional problems run in families, and often my patients felt more comfortable describing how they manifested themselves in previous generations. Doing so relieved the patients of an oppressive sense of guilt and responsibility. When I said, "You didn't cause this problem, but you can do something to correct it," they understood.

But patients might also respond to my "How can I help?" with "I don't know" or "I'm not even sure why I'm here." Some were unable to give up their inner fear. "My abdominal pain may be caused by cancer, and the doctors just have not been able to find it, despite four or five second opinions." Such patients weren't ready for psychotherapy. They were often under a somatic delusion, which is a fixed false belief. Because it is fixed, there is no point in challenging the patient's belief. If the patient seemed a bit uncertain about the suspicion of cancer or heart disease, I would ask, "When did this symptom first bother you?" When the patient responded, for example, "Five or six years ago," I would say, "What was going on at that time?"

If a patient said, "Sometimes my pain is so bad that I can't move," I'd ask, "What does that keep you from doing?" Then at this point the narrative could begin, and our focus on the symptom changed to what was happening in his or her life. For example, a patient might say, "Because of the diarrhea, friends and family have to come to my house. I'm bound to the porcelain. I can't go out." Once the patient had opened this door, I coaxed out the story. "Tell me more about that," or I'd say, "And then what happened?"

As I listened to the content of the story, I also paid close attention to nonverbal clues, to the tone and body language that accompanied the telling. Good poker players are experts at interpreting these clues. The first time an opponent adjusts her glasses or pulls on his ear, an expert will watch carefully what happens with that poker hand. If the opponent twists his wedding ring during a bluff, the next time he twists that ring, he is bluffing again. In the world of poker, these are known as "tells." What I learned from patients' "tells," or nonverbal clues, I would point out to the patient. For example, when a patient raised his voice, I would interrupt and ask, "Are you aware that you are raising your voice? Do you know what it means when you do that?"

"No," he or she almost invariably replied.

"It means you're feeling defensive," I'd say. "We need to find out why." Tears and blushes were obvious signs of sadness or anger in the first case and shame and anger in the second. I was also always on the lookout for what we call Freudian slips, or, verbal mistakes. If my patient said, "my father" when she meant "my husband," I would break in and say, "Let's talk about that."

Unconscious clues like these are shortcuts to emotions. Once I got that physiologic response, I was where I wanted to be. When the patient reached for a tissue and began to cry, or when the patient shook his fist in anger, I kept quiet. The patient had to say the next thing. Once the emotion and the narrative accompanying it had played out, the patient often said something that underscored the significance of the breakthrough. Many patients have gone through life thinking they could never lose control or never allow themselves to express anger. After going through that most daunting barrier to successful therapy, real work could begin. I reinforced the good start. "How does that make you feel to have expressed that?" Almost always, the patient would say something like, "Relieved. It's a weight off my shoulders. I've been carrying it for a long time."

Then, if it seemed appropriate, I would pat the patient's hand or shoulder. The empathy these gestures expressed was real. Because emotions are contagious, I felt an echo of what the patient was feeling. When people bared their souls or delved into loss and trauma, it was incredibly moving. I, myself, was sometimes the one reaching for that box of tissues.

At this point, when the patient was vulnerable and open, I would suggest we call in whomever accompanied them. After the spouse or parents or children got settled in my office, I would give a brief summary of what the patient said and the emotions accompanying it. "Tom became very angry about feeling left out when you became so involved with the children," I would say. "As he expressed his anger, he noticed that his headache disappeared. He then knew that there was an important connection between his repressed anger and his pain." Frequently the spouse would take his hand and look tenderly at him.

Chapter Nine
Profile Self-Confrontation

Each of us has within us a common enemy. It may have many different faces, but it always has a similar identity–the sense of alienation, of being incomplete, inauthentic, divorced from ourselves. We expend so much energy keeping our "dark side" locked away that we have little energy left over for love, joy, learning, and creativity. But, this is not a mandatory life sentence.

By recognizing and accepting our "dark side," that is, our feeling side, and truly experiencing it, we can release energy to fuel joy and transcendence.

When I was the only psychiatrist at Scott & White, I discovered the enormous value of video, thanks to one patient. This patient, Mrs. Irving, was whiny, dependent, and masochistic, and our therapy sessions were going poorly. To help us figure out why, I asked a colleague at Scott & White to videotape one of our therapy sessions. When we reviewed the tape, I saw that I was holding my right index finger to my lips, as if to shush Mrs. Irving. This was not lost on her. "Aha!" she accused. "You're trying to shut me up. But no wonder. Listen to my whining." Not long after, I read in a professional journal that Dr. Ian Alger, a psychoanalyst practicing in New York City, was using innovative video techniques in his practice, so I called him. He invited me to attend a workshop he was conducting for psychiatrists. I was elated.

Fifteen psychiatrists and clinical psychologists crowded into a small studio on Manhattan's Upper West Side. Playing on the video monitor was a tape of two people arguing. The man raised his voice and pointed at his wife. This was followed by a shot of Ian Alger talking to the couple: "Did you realize that you were raising your voice and pointing at your wife?" he asked.

"I didn't do that," the man replied. But watching the replay of the session, the husband could not avoid the truth. Alger showed his increasingly impressed colleagues several other ways he used video techniques to help patients gain insight. Among these were patients' soliloquies. Patients were allowed to describe themselves for three minutes and then review the tape and comment on how they felt.

But what really excited me was Alger's demonstration of what he called Profile Self-Confrontation. At first the image on the screen was visually confusing. There were two seemingly different individuals nose-to-nose, confronting each other; however, the screen was showing two sides of the same person. One camera was focused on the right side of the patient's face, the other camera was focused on the left side. The two profiles were then projected onto a screen, and the two sides of the one person were literally facing off. The right side was confronting the left side. It took several seconds to recognize that we were looking at the same person because the profiles were so different. One would look confident, the other frightened, one arrogant, the other sad. Without making any comment, Alger let us take this in. For me it triggered that powerful memory of seeing my left profile in the mirror in O'Connor's Men's Store when I was a young man in Rochester, Minnesota.

After giving us a couple of minutes to absorb the impact of the confronting profiles, Alger described the principle behind this therapeutic tool. It was an extension of what the great experimental psychologist Werner Wolff had pioneered with the use of still photography. In 1933, fifteen years before I bought my first suit, Werner Wolff started exploring human expressions. He studied the face, hands, gait, and voices of his subjects and said, "These experiments were designed to answer the question of whether the inner personality (the unconscious) is reflected in external behavior." He wondered whether people would even recognize their own forms of expressions and presented them recordings of their voices, pictures of their profiles, and pictures of their hands. Most could not identify themselves.

He also made full-face portraits of subjects from a combination of the left and right sides of the face. He split the full-face photographs and placed two left side profiles and two right side profiles together so that one full face contained two left sides and the other contained two right sides. The composites of the two right profiles were usually identified by the subjects as looking

110

like themselves, but full-face composites of the two left profiles were not generally recognized. The subjects frequently had strong feelings of aversion to them. This led Wolff to realize that the subjects had the most intense feelings about the unrecognized reflections of themselves and that intense self-judgment, according to Wolff "goes deeper into the personality. It is also strongly tinged with emotion and tinged toward positive or negative exaggeration. As a rule the unconscious self-judgment tends to idealize, and it is possible to show in a series of anamneses [recallings] that this idealization expresses the subconscious wishes of the subject."

He believed that the "wish image," if recognized, could lead to important insights about the person. The right profile composite reflected the conscious aspect of the person while the left profile composite was a reflection of the unconscious facets of the same person. Unlike Wolff's still photographs, Alger's technique captured changes in the profiles at the very moments the subjects experienced the emotion. His patients, too, were astonished when they saw the difference in their two profiles. Some even began spontaneous dialogues between the two sides.

When I returned from New York, I persuaded Scott & White's president, Olin Gober, to invest in the remaining equipment I needed in order to begin using Profile Self-Confrontation, or PSC. Gober, a cardiologist, was agreeably open to new ideas. Known as one of the most compassionate, thoughtful physicians around, a doctor who really listened to patients, he had supported my having our inpatients do painting and sculpture to aid in their diagnosis and treatment, so I was not surprised when he reacted favorably to my proposal. He even helped set up the equipment, using a former patient room as a studio. After we had figured out the lighting and camera angles, I insisted on being the guinea pig. My left profile troubled me, just as it had in O'Connor's in Rochester, but this time it was the other side that shocked me. "It's alarming to see the insufferable arrogance in my right profile," I confessed. With a sly smile, Olin Gober replied, "That bit of insight alone is well worth the price of the equipment." A line from Scottish poet Robert Burns, memorized in some distant high school English literature class, came to mind: "Oh wad some power the giftie gie

111

us/To see ourselves as others see us."

After that first experiment with Profile Self-Confrontation, I was hooked. Despite my own psychoanalysis, I had a mid-life crisis in my forties and gained thirty-five pounds. I had continued having occasional PSC sessions just to try to keep up with what was going on within my own psyche. At that time my left profile looked angry, and my right was fat and happy. In my fifties, my profiles evened out. I was thin with graying hair and beard. In my sixties I looked more depressed on my left side. At that time I had announced my retirement, and for almost two years I had to work through my feelings about patients accusing me of not caring. I worked through that crisis by writing poetry. I hadn't written a poem since the eighth grade when Miss Glendenning stopped our class and instructed us to look out the window and write a poem about the heavy snowfall. We all grumbled and then silence fell over the room. As I wrote my poem, I entered a "flow state" which lasted until the bell rang.

In my seventies, the evenness in my profiles returned. Doing the PSC helped me realize that the old man on the screen was really me. PSC has been an important source of insight for me all my life, starting quite by accident when I was seventeen and trying to buy a new suit.

Profile Self-Confrontation is an extremely valuable therapy, particularly for those patients who are prone to externalize or project conflicts. At Scott & White our technique of PSC was patterned after Ian Alger's. The patient sat in front of a television monitor while the therapist sat behind and to the side of the patient. The images were made by carefully balancing the lighting and the cameras. In this way even subtle changes in skin color were captured. The patient and I looked at the person's right and left profiles which were nose to nose on a screen in front of us. Most patients were struck instantly by the significant differences in their profiles, so I allowed two or three minutes for them to adjust to their profiles before they were asked to describe what they saw.

Almost without fail, the patient began on a positive note with

112

the right profile, and an initial negative reaction and aversion to the left profile. I then asked the patient to name the profiles. A typical response might be "nice guy" and "mean punk." The patient was then asked to develop a dialogue between the profiles. Often the responses resembled those of Wolff's subjects when viewing the posed photographs: "For the right side of the face: vivacious, robust, good-natured, extrovert, and on the left side, calm, inhibited, imaginative, malicious, introvert." There was almost always agreement between me and my patient about the perceived expressions of the profiles.

With this technique, we were able to view spontaneous changes and dramatic alterations in facial expression as the patient experienced various emotions. As these emotions played out, Wolff's "unconscious" side frequently became "conscious" and this had substantial, enduring therapeutic benefit for my patients.

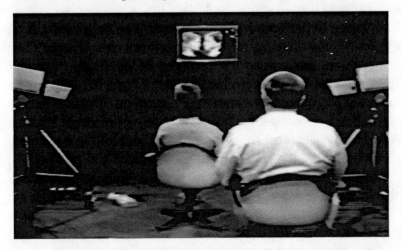

Illustration No. 9: In our studio at Scott & White, the patient, in background, is taped with two cameras, each focused on one side of the face. The physician is seated behind the woman.

Over the years, I saw PSC work dramatically with patient after patient suffering from a variety of debilitating emotional disorders. For some the technique proved too powerful. They found the direct delivery of insight too disturbing, so they refused to

113

participate. But most patients were willing to make the effort and brave the vulnerability and experienced dramatic short-term relief and lasting improvement.

Profile Self-Confrontation is, I believe, one of the most effective superhighways to repressed emotions. It literally helps patients face the truth, which is difficult and painful to do. We think the person we present to the world is the true us, when, in fact, this persona is only half of the truth. Most humans want to be better than we are, but most of us have settled for a public image that we protect fiercely.

Profile Self-Confrontation: The Magic Box

Until Canadian psychiatrist Norman Doidge, M.D., wrote *The Brain that Changes Itself*, the scientific community believed neurons in the brain and spinal cord could not regenerate, so recovery from injury to the central nervous system was impossible. It was a fixed system—fixed at birth. But this is not true. Doidge's book demonstrates many scientific examples of seemingly miraculous cures affected by the brain healing itself. Now the belief is that the brain can change or "rearrange" based on thinking; learning and acting can change the brain's anatomy or physical structure. A review by *The New York Times* of this best-selling book states, "This book straddles the gap between science and self-help." In the book Doidge describes a patient with phantom limb pain, a phenomenon which has always troubled healers. How can a nonexistent arm have disabling chronic pain? The answer is that the pain must exist in the brain.

Dr. Doidge writes about a research technique to trick the brain: The researcher built a cake-sized box with arm-sized holes in each end and placed a mirror on edge in the middle of the box. The box was open on the top so that the subject could look down into it. The sufferer who was having pain in his phantom left arm placed the right arm in the box and tilted his head so he could see the mirror image of his left arm. Then by moving his right arm, it appeared to him that he was moving his left arm. That movement registered in his brain map, and the pain promptly disappeared,

114

but it reappeared as soon as he looked away.

The subject was instructed to take the box home and to repeat the process. After several days of practicing this exercise, he lost the pain for good without having to look into the box. It was like a magical removal of the pain in the phantom limb. Dr. Doidge writes that our brains are plastic like the children's clay Playdoh and can be malleable.

For forty years I have used PSC with amazing success to remove disabling somatic (physical) symptoms. These symptoms are caused by repressed unconscious conflicts and the goal is to cure the symptoms. I always wondered how Profile Self-Confrontation actually worked. What could explain this phenomenon? Now I have compelling evidence with Doidge's research that PSC is its own magic box. A respected group of neuroplasticians are doing research on how the brain changes itself. I hope this group will do research on the enormous potential PSC has for healing the brain.

When viewing both profiles nose to nose, the subject sees significant differences between the left and right profiles. The right looks familiar, but the left looks so different that the subject often refuses to recognize it as his or her face. However, when the subject names them and begins a conversation between the two sides, the facial expression changes. The left profile has for too long been repressed, but when the brain sees the left profile changing, then the brain changes as well. Insight allows the repressed unconscious conflicts to become conscious, and the disabling symptoms disappear. It is often helpful to subjects to repeat the PSC to cement their insights and to allow them to see the dramatic changes in their facial expressions. The patients no longer look ill.

Noting that the scientific method requires scientists to be ever mindful of the danger of the observer influencing the results of an experiment, Harvard psychology professor, Daniel Gilbert, asked in his book *Stumbling on Happiness*:

> If views are acceptable only when they are credible, and if they are credible only when they are based on facts, then how do we achieve positive views of ourselves and our experiences? How do we manage to think of ourselves as great drivers, talented lovers and brilliant chefs

when the facts of our lives include a pathetic parade of dented cars, disappointed partners, and deflated soufflés? The answer is simple. We cook the facts.

How does this work? William James, the great nineteenth-century American psychologist, described how feelings follow action. In modern terms a way to understand James' explanation is to imagine that a car headed in the opposite direction veers into your lane. You skillfully avoid a head-on collision by steering to the right, taking your foot off the accelerator and holding the car steady on the shoulder. You may be remotely aware of your icy calm. As your vehicle comes gently to a stop, you are so over-whelmed by fear that you shake. Yet the danger has passed. Had you felt an incapacitating level of fear during the crisis, you would not have been able to steer your car to safety. You would prob-ably be dead, or at least seriously injured. Your feelings followed your action, and it was a good thing that they did. Likewise, once patients confront their conscious controlling right profiles and un-conscious feeling left profiles, their previously repressed feelings can follow.

Facial Action Coding System

Dr. Paul Ekman, professor of psychology at the University of California at San Francisco School of Medicine, is an internation-ally recognized expert on facial expression and emotion. He made an analysis of the muscle movements involved in expressing feel-ings, then compiled his findings in what he called the Facial Ac-tion Coding System. Using trained actors, he conducted an in-teresting experiment that demonstrated a remarkable relationship between expression and emotion. Rather than telling the actors to "look frightened" or "look happy," he instructed them to move certain facial muscles in certain ways. Without being aware that they were doing so, the actors assumed frightened expressions, happy expressions, angry expressions, and so on. Each time the actor moved facial muscles in a certain feigned mood, he experi-enced the corresponding feeling.

116

Ekman's subjects were not viewing themselves in a mirror or on videotape. Instead, they were experiencing these emotions kinesthetically. The changes in their muscles produced them. Human beings are strongly sight-oriented, and we're fixated on faces. That is how we pick up the emotional cues we need to interrelate, and that is why emotions are contagious. We walk into a party, see someone who looks sad, and pick up that mood. Or, if we are feeling upbeat and smile warmly, our morose fellow guest may "catch" our mood. On the basis of his research, Ekman developed a test called "The Relived Emotional Status Exam," which I combined with Profile Self-Confrontation to help patients relive emotions. (See Appendix A.) When the physiology of the repressed emotion is released and realized, the patient can see, know, and own that emotion. Insight follows.

In 1859 Dinah Mulock Craik wrote in *A Life for a Life:* "Oh the comfort—the inexpressible comfort—of feeling *safe* with a person having neither to weigh thoughts nor measure words, but pouring them all right out, just as they are, chaff and grain together; certain that a faithful hand shall take and sift them, keep what is worth the keeping, and then with the breath of kindness, blow the rest away."

In PSC I could exercise a "breath of kindness." The right profile was the chaff, the public persona, and the left side was the grain, the part we need to confront for true insight to occur. In an individual who was experiencing emotional or chronic physical problems, psychological defenses protect this left side, covering it over, packing it down, encasing it in the psychological equivalent of concrete. A person in that position cannot get through these defenses without help, and that is precisely what Profile Self-Confrontation offers.

Profile Self-Confrontation Healing

Compassionate listening of the same sort my father and his colleagues practiced in the early twentieth century was my single key to Profile Self-Confrontation. It was straightforward and easy to master technically, but it worked only if I were wholly present, engaged, and emotionally connected with the patient. When I welcomed patients to our first appointment, I would shake hands and look at their facial expression. Touching the patients and noticing their dress gave me important clues. One morning I opened my office door to a thirty-five year-old man. Most people stood up, introduced themselves, and shook my hand. He did not. When I leaned down to shake his hand, he apologized for the grease. "I work in a filling station," he explained. Embroidered above the pocket of his blue-striped shirt was "Ben's Shell Service," and on the other side, "Ben, Jr." When I asked how I could be of help, he took a deep breath and exhaled. Then he took another.

"I'm having terrible heart problems," Ben, Jr. said. "My heart races. I have numbness and tingling in my arms, and sometimes I get spasms—cramps in my hands. I don't know why the cardiologist sent me to you."

I did not have to be Sherlock Holmes to deduce my new patient's problem. It became apparent to me immediately. Most patients dress up for an appointment with a physician. By coming in his dirty work clothes, Ben, Jr. conveyed his self-image. He saw himself as Ben, Sr.'s grease monkey. He had a hostile and dependent relationship with a father who had discouraged him from developing his own identity. Although he was furious about being dependent, the patient had repressed his anger, expressing it indirectly through his sighing and hyperventilation. The hyperventilation lowered his carbon dioxide level, which made him anxious. The anxiety brought on his other distressing physiologic symptoms, including the racing of his heart, his numbing and tingling, and the cramping of his muscles.

I could have prescribed medicine to treat his anxiety, but I have always considered anxiety a symptom. I wanted to deal with the underlying cause, so I scheduled a PSC session. As the twin video cameras recorded his images, Ben, Jr. saw his angry right profile and his frightened left profile. He named the right one "Ben" and the left one "Stupid Jerk." Immediately, he recognized how difficult it was for him to begin a dialogue between his two sides. "Ben has to be in control," he observed. He understood that resolving his inner conflict meant allowing Stupid Jerk to speak, so he began to allow his left profile to challenge the right.

Because these inner dialogues were so helpful to him, Ben Jr. and I did three PSC sessions. He shared them with his long-term fiancée, but not his parents. She urged him to allow her to call his parents and set up a chance for the four of them to view the tapes together. Finally, he relented. Later, when the family began watching the three PSC sessions together, they began sharing emotions. Two weeks later Ben, Jr. came in for another appointment. He stood up to greet me. He wore slacks and a pressed shirt. His fingernails were clean. "The Stupid Jerk is better," he announced. Profile Self-Confrontation had taught Ben to deal directly with his emotions. Armed with this new ability and insight, he could begin to resolve his identity crisis and dependency issues. And he had not needed anti-anxiety medication.

Relived Emotional Assessment

Usually during one of the Profile Self-Confrontation sessions, I conducted what's called a Relived Emotional Assessment of seven basic emotions: happiness, contempt, fear, anger, disgust, sadness, and relief. The assessment began with "happiness," which was usually (but not always) the least threatening. Making sure my patient was looking at the monitor I'd say, "For the first fifteen seconds, just empty your mind of all thoughts, feelings and emotions." Then I'd ask the patient to remember a time when he or she felt a strong sense of happiness. "Tell me about that time," I said. "Now, go back into that time and try to feel the happiness that you felt then. When you begin to feel the happiness again, let the feeling grow, and when you are feeling the happiness as strongly as you can, say, 'I feel happy.' "

Following that reply, I had the patient repeat that declaration twice, each time with more feeling. Then I instructed him to gather in all the happiness he had ever experienced, express it in his face and body until he felt the emotion as strongly as he could and repeat, "I am happy."

After resting for fifteen seconds, I asked the patient to rank the feeling of happiness he just experienced on a scale of one to

119

eight. I'd ask, "Did you feel the most happiness the first, second, or third time you said, 'I am happy!' " Then, I asked if he felt any other emotions when he was saying, "I feel happy!" Did he experience contempt, fear, anger, disgust, or sadness? If the patient answered affirmatively to any of these, I had him rank the strength of that accompanying feeling on a scale of one to eight. The answers were usually remarkably revealing. We would take a break and then repeat the process, this time with the next emotional state—contempt. We continued in a similar manner with all the emotional states.

Most patients tended to inhibit certain feelings selectively. For example, a patient might be able to express sadness, but not anger or fear. On noticing anger in his left profile, one of my patients saw his right profile smile. "That's exactly what I do," he declared. "I feel anger, and then I smile. It's as if I'm inviting more abuse. It's like I enjoy being a doormat." Such information represented true clinical breakthroughs. When that happened, I affirmed their value. "That's a very significant insight," I'd say. "It's important that you understand what's happening here."

I thought it good practice to give approval, encouragement, and affirmation for this hard work, but to resist the temptation to make observations. Jumping in with an "ah-ha!" followed by an explanation ("Now we can see that your father did this or that, and the same thing is happening with your boss!") seemed to rob the patient of experiencing the breakthrough on an emotional and physiologic level. The patient needed to set the pace and to own the insights.

Some patients simply did not have the words to talk about feelings. This condition, called alexithymia, is fairly common in areas of the country where emotional control is considered a virtue, even an essential life skill. God-fearing, hardworking, perfectionist people are frequently alexithymic. "They won't say shit if they have a mouthful" goes the coarse but apt saying. For example, in less congested regions, I rarely hear a car honk, whereas in large cities a car is considered disabled if its horn stops blowing. If I corner a controlled city person and confront him, it might provoke an angry outburst, while the man from the smaller town will give me a tight little smile and say, "I don't appreciate that." (But be warned. The driver may say this just before he punches out your lights.)

One patient, whom I will call Mrs. Cannon because she was at war with her husband and children, was admitted to our inpatient unit because she had threatened suicide. Her husband knew she had a gun, but she refused to tell him where it was. All this was complicated by her background. Her grandfather had been a legendary and flamboyant West Texas businessman. As his favorite, she was used to getting her way.

Mrs. Cannon was furious at her husband and children. Fearful that she would kill them as well as herself, her local internist, who had been treating her for depression and eating disorders, referred her to me at Scott & White, even though Temple, Texas, was more than three hundred miles from her home. When I met Mrs. Cannon, she impressed me as an articulate woman with pressured speech. She was tall and rangy and chain-smoked throughout the interview. She made it clear that seeing a psychiatrist was the idea of her local doctor and of her husband, but she did admit that, "My anger is driving everyone away." To make matters more serious, she had told them she had a gun. She explained, "But I think I said that to let them know I was miserable, alone, and that I needed help." She recognized she was mentally ill and agreed to enter our psychiatric unit.

Once she was admitted psychological tests substantiated my initial impression that she had a borderline personality disorder. On good days she was highly neurotic, on bad ones, psychotic. She participated enthusiastically in art therapy, but she left herself out of her paintings. Her ego was so poorly developed that she could not see herself as an authentic person. During our initial Profile Self-Confrontation session, she immediately looked at the left profile and said, "I'm a terrified little girl." This was a part of herself she had never seen. She normally came across as demanding and powerful, shouting, insisting that things be done her way.

Then she looked at her right profile. "Oh, my God! The anger!" Suddenly, she had an insight. "I'm not angry at everybody else,"

121

she said. "I'm just trying to keep people away from my help-less side." Shortly thereafter Mrs. Cannon's husband and grown children visited her; their reunion was moving. They examined her paintings appreciatively and thoughtfully. They viewed the videotapes of the PSC sessions and discussed the insights they gleaned from them. Mrs. Cannon's family had never seen that vulnerable side of her, but now they recognized that her anger was a defense. It was not their fault and they did not have to take it personally. That was not always the outcome, however.

Another patient I'll call Inez came to Scott & White com-plaining of excruciating, disabling pain in her left flank. After the examinations and tests conducted by our Department of In-ternal Medicine showed no underlying pathology, her physician requested a psychiatry consultation. She was admitted to our unit. The pain had begun four years earlier, immediately after her son's death from cancer. The son had asked the family not to tell Inez about his condition. He sought help at Houston's renowned M.D. Anderson Cancer Center where he underwent surgery, radiation therapy, and chemotherapy without ever informing his mother. When Inez finally became alarmed at his appearance ("His hair fell out, and he lost all that weight," she explained), he confessed, saying he had wanted to spare her feelings.

Although never having been out of Falls County, Texas, be-fore, she drove to Houston and camped out in his hospital room. "I never left him," she told me. He died with her sitting there with her left side facing him. It was the same side on which she expe-rienced the pain. During the Profile Self-Confrontation, I asked Inez if she was angry with her son's excluding her. "Not angry," she said, "disappointed."

Inez was born in 1919 on a Central Texas farm. She was the oldest child in a large family. "We were poor," she recalled, pro-nouncing it "purr." "We didn't have everything we wanted and a lot of times not everything we needed." During the Great Depres-sion the family eked out a living as farmers. They lived in a shot-gun shack without electricity or running water. Inez remembered her father as an angry and sometimes violent man ("He would always blow his top.") who died from a stroke when she was fourteen. Her only source of security had been her church. "I knew that Jesus cared for me," she said. Because her help was needed on the farm, Inez finished only the eighth grade. She got married at fifteen "to an older man. He was twenty-seven." They raised three children. Her husband died six months after her son. Without the support of her husband and son, Inez's insecurity overwhelmed her, and she became dependent on her pain medication.

When I asked Inez to relive her sadness, she said she could not. I asked her if she had ever said good-bye to her son and she replied, "No." I urged her to say good-bye, to express her grief, explaining that then she might lose her pain, but as her left profile began to show grief, Inez closed her eyes. Try as I might to persuade her to open her eyes and confront her grief, she refused. When she did open her eyes, her profiles revealed no emotion. She terminated the session saying, "My son is all I have left." She then confessed that she had lost her faith in Jesus when her son died. She left the unit the next day with the plan to return to her physician and continue the pain medication. With most patients, PSC is a powerful tool, but in some cases, particularly those with refractory pain problems, (pain problems that don't respond to medical treatment) patients would rather live with their pain than give up the defense.

Although a small number of patients might resist PSC's effectiveness, in my experience, the combination of PSC and the Relived Emotional Assessment was the most effective technique for achieving a fairly fast breakthrough to insight in patients disabled by pain or other symptoms caused by repressed conflicts. The method was also especially useful with two disparate groups of patients who were the most challenging to other clinicians: those who were psychologically unsophisticated and the opposite, those who knew a lot about psychology, perhaps having years of therapy and even academic study in the field. The latter were people who protected their defenses by being bright, controlling, and adept at intellectualizing. That was true whether they were experiencing acute physical symptoms such as irritable bowel syndrome, chest pain, or vague, ill-defined malaise, fatigue and anhedonia, the inability to enjoy life.

For some, one PSC session was enough to take them where they needed to go. They viewed the left profile (unconscious) and the right profile (conscious, public persona), and for the first time these two sides were able to communicate. The patient was at the place where god and the devil were on speaking terms.

A patient for whom PSC was especially gratifying was a Mrs. Holtzer, the seventy-two year-old widow of a local businessman. She was completing detoxification from barbiturate dependency for the third time, and the nursing staff questioned the decision to continue inpatient treatment for her. Their argument that it would be futile thinly concealed their underlying reason—they could not stand her. After her husband died six years earlier, Mrs. Holtzer had become an angry, bitterly complaining, drug-dependent person who totally alienated herself from everyone, including the nurses and her fellow patients. Although she had two daughters living nearby, they refused to visit her or to be involved, yet again, in planning her discharge. "After Daddy's death, she became an impossible witch," one daughter explained. I reviewed all of this with Mrs. Holtzer and urged her to stay for a trial of PSC, suggesting that she might benefit from looking at her profiles. Maybe then she would be able to see, literally, that her anger was preventing her from dealing with her unresolved grief about her husband's death. To my surprise, she agreed.

As soon as she saw her profiles nose to nose, her attitude changed. "Look at the anger on the right," she exclaimed. "And, dear God, look at the grief on the left! I'm fighting myself, not everybody else." Seeing the physical manifestation of her unresolved grief unlocked the emotion itself. Immediately, we both focused on her left profile, and I suggested that it was time to say goodbye to her husband. She shook her head no, then paused. Her voice filled with tears, and she said, "Dear heart, it is time for me to say goodbye." She sat motionless for a few moments and then in a soft voice said, "Goodbye."

She began sobbing. Her head dropped leaving only patches of white hair bobbing up and down on the monitor. Moans and screams punctuated the sobs, but after a few minutes, Mrs. Holtzer lifted her head and studied her profiles again. Her anger was gone, and her grief had softened to sadness. She asked me if her daughters could come watch the PSC tape with her. They did. After a lot of hugging and crying, they all left together. On follow-up Mrs. Holtzer continued to function well and to enjoy a close relationship with her family. Ten years later, she died in our hospital following a stroke. Her daughters were at her bedside.

For patients like Mrs. Holtzer, I scheduled a follow-up visit a week or so later to see how they were doing. If the somatic symptoms were gone or the patient seemed to have come to terms with the issues that caused the emotional distress, one additional session was sufficient. Typically, the patient would express gratitude and recapitulate the major insight. "Thank you so much, doctor! I never realized I had so much trouble expressing sadness." Or, "Things are going so much better at home. My daughter understands that my anger really wasn't at her."

Reactions like these were profoundly gratifying and affirming, both intellectually and emotionally. They reinforced my conviction that helping the patient unlock the feeling was key to resolving the symptom. One reason I treasure those moments is because the course of therapy was not always that smooth and straightforward. The highway to emotion can contain twists, turns, and steep hills. In some cases, a patient would tell me that he or she thought another PSC would be helpful. For example, one woman who was having trouble grieving about her alcoholic husband's death, might, during the first session, get in touch with her anger at his abuse, but might need another session to access her sadness at the loss of the relationship as it was and as it never had a chance to be.

For Ben, Jr., whose case I described earlier, PSC was the only way he could experience anger, sadness, and disgust. Repeating the technique was essential to his progress in psychotherapy. The anger at his father came out in the first session. The second session brought forth his disgust at what he had and had not done with his life. The third enabled him to get in touch with his sadness at never having had his own dream, never having had a sense

125

of what he wanted to accomplish.

Emotionally ill patients look sick, just as patients with cancer or multiple sclerosis do. Since the sick look is so striking, it must serve an important evolutionary function. If one individual tells another, "I'm sick," the immediate response is to search the face of the claimant closely. "But you don't look sick!" may be the rejoinder. But more often the response will be, "I can see you're not well. Let me help."

In 1982, a young woman I will call Emily attempted suicide by sticking her head in an oven and turning on the gas. Discovering her before she had lost consciousness, her mother brought her to Scott & White. We admitted her as an inpatient and began a course of therapy that included individual sessions, group therapy, and PSC.

When I took Emily's history, she told me about several previous psychiatric hospitalizations she had undergone. Explosive conflicts with her mother punctuated Emily's chaotic home life. Although she had graduated from college and worked as a translator, she still lived with her parents. She looked vulnerable, fragile, and disorganized. Above all, she looked sick. I diagnosed her as suffering from borderline personality disorder. In order to survive she would have to separate from her highly dysfunctional family. The therapeutic goal we agreed on was to help her get over her grief. Emily was clearly an excellent candidate for PSC. The sessions accelerated the progress she had made through her paintings, which could be wry or wrenching. In one painting she depicted herself in a red miniskirt, dragging a ball and chain.

The day before she was discharged, Emily showed me the edited version of her PSC tapes. (Illustrations Nos. 10-14) They ranged from March fifteenth to June eighth. Commenting on the first, she described her right and left profiles as "not looking remotely alike." She saw her right profile "holding me back. It wouldn't let the anger out," she said. "The left side is mad. The right side doesn't know anything. It's a timid little man. The left eye is crying, but not the right." (As strange as it seems, that sometimes happens.) Looking at the April twenty-first tape, Em-

126

ily said her left side was "madder." She said she thought it was beginning to understand what was going on, and her right side was sad. "That was the point in therapy where I began to see what was happening to me. And both sides are crying."

By looking at the tape recorded four weeks later, Emily was able to deal with the fact that her mother had her own emotional problems. She had rejected Emily because of these issues, not because Emily was "evil" or "a bad seed." "The left side looks heartbroken and filled with grief," Emily remarked. "The right side looks stronger. Both sides look even, but the left side looks tired." After more sessions and insight, Emily interpreted the tape-recorded May twenty-fifth this way:

> The profiles are more even, the same. They're not angry anymore. For the first time in her life, she looks like a person who knows what she's doing. One side doesn't misrepresent the other. The right always misrepresented the left. The left looks older, more whole. And both sides are crying. It's like a whole person, not divided anymore.

Then, looking at her June eighth tape Emily observed, "My profiles match. They're happy, whole. Seems like a miracle. This

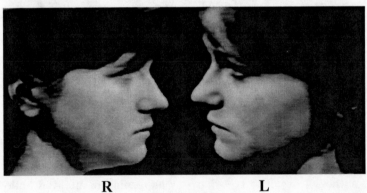

R   L

Illustration No. 10: In her first profile, with left in every instance being the right side of the face and right being the left side of her face, Emily commented that they did not look remotely alike. She saw her right profile "holding me back. It wouldn't let the anger out." The left side, she saw as mad, saying, "The right side doesn't know anything. It's a timid little man. The left eye is crying, but not the right."

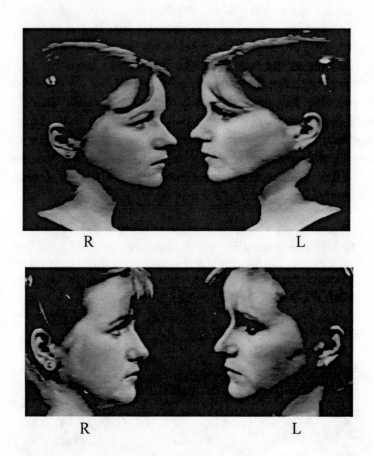

R   L

R   L

Illustrations No. 11 and 12: Looking at the April twenty-first tape, above top, Emily said her left side was "madder." She said she thought it was beginning to understand what was going on, and her right side was sad. "That was the point where I began to see what was happening to me. And both sides are crying," she said. Four weeks later, in photo directly above, Emily said she was able to deal with the fact that her own mother had her own emotional problems. Her mother had rejected her as evil and a bad seed. "The left side looks heartbroken and filled with grief," she said. "The right side looks stronger. Both sides look even, but the left side looks tired."

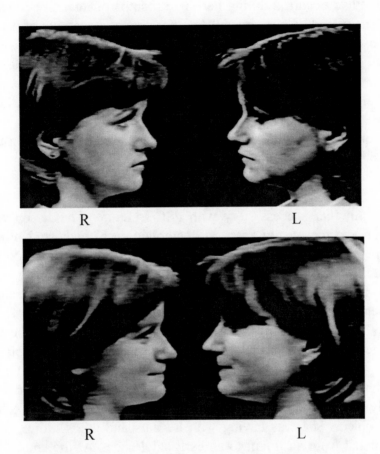

R   L

R   L

Illustrations No. 13 and 14: On May twenty-fifth, shown at top above, Emily described her profiles as more even, more the same, not angry any more. Both sides are crying because she believes she looks like a whole person, with the right no longer misinterpreting the left. Above, looking at her June eighth tape, Emily declared herself happy and whole.

is the only visible evidence of how much better I am. I'm the glowing picture of health. I know I won't go crazy, and that's a big deal. I feel confident in my abilities now. I feel irrepressible. I see a difference in my profiles, but it's a happy difference."

When I showed Emily's tapes to Hans Selye who believed

"sick people look sick," he could see the dramatic facial changes that had occurred during her three months of intensive psychotherapy and he exclaimed, "Another dramatic example of what I observed in medical school!"

Emily left the unit eager to take her place as a very talented player in the game of life. She got engaged to an English writer, and we arranged for her to continue her psychotherapy at London's renowned Tavistock Clinic. In 2006, I contacted Emily to request her permission to include the photos of her PSC in this book. Although some of her concerns have returned, she is happily married and is so much better than when she started therapy.

Another success story with PSC is Lauren Henderson who came to me twenty years ago complaining of malaise. Nothing specific had been wrong, but she had no zest for life. Nothing seemed worth the effort. Although she routinely won recognition as a top teacher, she had lost interest in her profession. I treated her as an outpatient. Lauren had grown up in a legendary Texas dynasty. Her identity was totally tied up in her family and the role she played in it, especially the face she presented to the public.

We began with traditional weekly therapy sessions in which she gave me her history, showed me her drawings of her family constellation, looked at family photographs, and discussed the problems she was having with her husband and children, who ranged from an infant to an early adolescent. At the end of the second session, I suggested we do a PSC with a Relived Emotional Status Exam.

When she focused on her angry, confused, hidden left side, she experienced a powerful breakthrough. The following week, we repeated the process and then devoted the next four sessions to exploring the material we had unearthed. Over these weeks, Lauren repeatedly viewed the tapes, sometimes at home, sometimes with me. Her internal conflict subsided, and she recovered her energy and enjoyment of life. All it took was three months of weekly outpatient sessions and no medication.

A few years later, I ran into Lauren. She told me how much the PSCs had done for her, how the experience had turned her life around, and she asked if we could repeat them. Although she seemed in good emotional health, I agreed. We arranged follow-up sessions, and once those were complete and she had reviewed the tapes, she said that was all she needed. She thanked me. I never saw her again as a patient. The account Lauren sent me following our last appointment was so affirming to me professionally, and such a clear and moving expression of the benefits of Profile Self-Confrontation that with her permission I include it in Appendix C. It is so eloquently written that I wish I could credit her by name, but Lauren has asked me to keep her identity confidential.

Profile Self-Confrontation worked with one of those rare patients who elicited an immediate response of fear in me. Dr. Adam Clark, an experienced gastroenterologist, referred a sixty-three year-old minister to me. Calvin arrived for our first meeting wearing a plaid cotton shirt, a bolo tie, blue Sans-a-Belt pants, and scuffed brown shoes with white cotton socks. He glared at the abstract paintings on my office walls. His jaws worked like he was chewing tough meat. His wife of forty-one years, Mary, was with him, and her eyes were begging him to accept help.

I had already read Dr. Clark's referral notes: "Patient's current abdominal pain occurred first seventeen years ago when Calvin Jr. was killed in a one-car accident. Patient had a laparotomy because patient described the pain as a crab eating his bowels, and he wanted it removed. The notes read, "laparotomy, negative. Pain returned three months ago. All GI (gastrointestinal) tests negative." I was wary of Calvin, but I also empathized with him. I could imagine his routine of tending his congregation, taking countless trips to hospitals, nursing homes, and cemeteries, and giving sermon after sermon on God's love. He was always the caregiver. He had been taught that each adversity was a spiritual challenge, and that the Almighty would never present him with a challenge that he could not meet. It became obvious to me that he never had been, and never could be, dependent. Now that his pain prevented him from working, Calvin felt useless. All his self-worth was wrapped up in his being caring, responsible, and useful, and his hope that Dr. Adam Clark and our great multi-specialty healing center would cure him had vanished.

I assumed my customary therapeutic position, sitting in a chair next to Calvin. I never let my desk come between my patient and me. Suddenly, the lights went out, plunging my windowless office into complete darkness. Calvin jumped up and demanded angrily, "Now what, doctor?" I could feel his towering presence in the darkness. "Well, I'm an old Eagle Scout," I replied, "always prepared." I opened my desk drawer, retrieved a candle and a book of matches. Lighting the candle, I tilted it to pour a puddle of wax on a low table next to Calvin. He sat down and stared at the soft, flickering light, which glinted off his steel-rimmed glasses.

Calvin sat back in his chair, uncrossed his legs, and gave a deep sigh. My fear disappeared. Candlelight sparkled on the tears spilling down his face. Then came the sobs, deep, deep sobs. Suddenly the lights came on. A lightning strike had caused Scott & White's first power outage in thirty years. I called for Mary to return to my office. She looked at her husband's face and cried, "The pain is gone." And he said, "Yes." He agreed to a PSC session the next day.

Non-verbal cues had made Calvin's repressed anger apparent to me at our first meeting. Calvin had to encounter his grief over the loss of his son, which he did the next day during his PSC. He showed the videotape of the session to his wife in my office and then took it home where they played it many times. A month later Calvin called to cancel our scheduled follow-up. "I'm doing much better," he explained.

Non-verbal clues signaling potential loss of control were, for me, much easier to detect with PSC than with other psychotherapeutic methods. For one thing, both the patient and I are focused on how the patient's face looks, as much as on what he or she says. (Consider the difference between this and the now largely abandoned practice of having the patient lie on a chaise lounge while the analyst sits in a chair behind the head of the chaise lounge taking notes.) On those rare occasions when patients appeared deeply conflicted by the PSC, they closed their eyes, turned away or got up and left. I then turned off the cameras and continued the

132

session face to face. "Obviously, you had a significant reaction," I would say. "Let's talk about that."

Once, I encountered a whole group of patients who had this sort of reaction. As part of the research project that Paul Ekman and I undertook, we involved a group of twenty chronic alcoholic men from the Scott & White outpatient alcohol program. With each patient, our team conducted a Relived Emotional Status Examination during a PSC. When asked to relive an experience when they were angry, six of the twenty got up from their chairs and terminated the session. None of the remainder could relive any anger at all. Most reported that they had experienced intense anger when drunk, but never when sober.

Mrs. Jackson was a highly disturbed woman in her early forties. She had been in and out of most of the psychiatric hospitals in Texas, including several stints in our unit at Scott & White. She cut herself compulsively with knives and razors when she was home, or with something like the spring from the inside of a toilet-paper holder when she was institutionalized. On a previous admission, she had sliced tendons in her foot so badly that she required surgery to repair them.

Normally, I did not attempt psychotherapy with a patient so explosively disturbed. This was one case where I knew drugs were clearly indicated. I preferred putting patients on high doses of selective serotonin re-uptake inhibitors, such as Zoloft, to defuse their anger, but she refused any medication. I conducted two PSC sessions—not to get her in touch with her feelings because they were spilling out all over the place, but to recreate the psychiatric equivalent of a "Hail Mary Pass" in football. It seemed to be our only chance. Tellingly, in the first session, Mrs. Jackson did not recognize her left side as herself. Furthermore, in creative therapy, her drawings and paintings dealt with surgeries in which part of her body was cut away.

We did a second PSC, with similar results. She could not integrate herself. She told me she was empty, that there was nothing there to integrate. Although we had Mrs. Jackson in seclusion, she managed to cut herself again. A member of the cleaning crew had brought a cart into Mrs. Jackson's room. Along with sponges and brushes was a putty knife. While the housekeeper's back was turned, Mrs. Jackson deftly and surreptitiously pilfered the knife and hid it. That evening she sliced her thighs and calves, cutting deep into her muscles and requiring more reconstructive surgery.

When he was notified, her husband, who had not visited her once since she was admitted, became outraged, hired a lawyer, and sued us for negligence. He eventually won the case, but the court awarded him only a dollar. The PSC tapes we screened for the jury demonstrated not only how disturbed Mrs. Jackson was, but also how hard we had attempted to connect with her and protect her. Even when she did get her hands on a knife, Mrs. Jackson had never been a danger to our staff or me. Her anger and destructiveness were focused inside, rather than out. Nonetheless, seeing the damage she did to herself was very upsetting to us all. We desperately wanted to get her to stop hurting herself, and the fact that she could be so inventive and devious in her compulsion to continue harming herself raised the specter of violence as a consequence of loss of control.

I have never had a patient who deteriorated or regressed following PSC, and I have never felt threatened by a patient during one of these sessions. I am convinced that this was not a consequence of my physical stature. The technique itself seemed protective to both patient and therapist.

Adele Morrow was a fifty-year-old woman from a nearby town. She felt lifeless, without any energy, and at times had suicidal thoughts. Her Scott & White internist felt she needed a psychiatric evaluation, so I admitted her to the psychiatric unit. When I first met her, I was surprised by her appearance. She looked extremely competent and denied feeling depressed or having suicidal thoughts. Adele said she felt extremely confident about much of her life, but had no energy left. She was the one who could be counted on to bring an excellent cake, everyone's favorite cake, to the church bake sale or to organize friends to cook for a family when the mother was sick or recovering from childbirth. She wore herself out taking care of everyone, and they loved her for it. When she showed up at our psychiatric unit, her main complaints were exhaustion and depression. She had mentioned suicide. My mentor, Howard Rome, had taught me that suicide was usually homicidal anger turned inward. I recognized that the object of therapy would be to help her recognize the roots of her anger and to enable her to access that rage so that she could deal with it appropriately.

What struck me during our first PSC session was that Mrs. Morrow's right profile looked supremely competent. Here was a leader who could handle any situation that arose and who could be the Rock of Gibraltar for her family and friends. I would have voted for her for president. The left profile looked crushingly sad. In my decades of using this technique, I had seldom come across a more asymmetrical face.

It took Mrs. Morrow a few minutes to recognize what was so obvious to me. As soon as she said, "I see the sadness," she began sobbing. We talked about what she felt and scheduled another session for the following day. The second session was an accelerated version of the first. When Mrs. Morrow examined her left profile she said, "I don't look so sad." Then she began sobbing. We did the Relived Emotional Status Examination, focusing on anger. That was when she told me about her husband's rejection. After she'd had a hysterectomy, her husband declared that he was never going to have sex with her again because she was "no longer a woman." She was so angry that she fantasized killing him. His rejection brought back her emotionally barren childhood. She never remembered receiving any love from anyone until she married her husband with whom she felt sexually competent and loved. As I asked her to relive her anger, she began screaming her rage. She raised the middle finger of her right hand, shook it at the monitor and began sobbing. I thought that Mrs. Morrow could take those insights and run, but the evening after that second Profile Self-Confrontation, four of her women friends visited her. They told

135

her that they could not understand why she was in the hospital. They wanted their old, competent Adele back. And they won. She checked out the next day. I never saw her again.

With most inpatients I would conduct a PSC session every week. Before the patient was discharged, he or she would edit the tapes, condensing them into a series of two-minute clips from each week. The patient would review this "director's cut" with me and discuss the changes in their profiles over the course of the intensive therapy. This almost always produced an additional level or insight, the "ah-ha!" breakthrough. Patients were amazed by the profound changes in their facial expression from one session to the next. "I don't look sick anymore!" one declared. Another announced, "It's like plastic surgery." Over time our repeated PSC sessions documented patients' progression from sick to well, and that evolution showed clearly in their faces.

Profile Self-Confrontation, combined with the adjunct of the Relived Emotional Status Examination, was effective, efficient, and safe. Those patients who experienced the physiologic release of powerful emotions were relieved of the weight of their previously repressed feelings. Those who could not tolerate experiencing and expressing these feelings would elect to continue ignoring them or covering them up.

This therapy, in my opinion, was not only effective for my patients, but also cost-effective for the health system. Even drug treatment for my patients with psychiatric disorders required professional time, monitoring for side-effects and other follow-up visits, not to mention the price of the medications themselves. Profile Self-Confrontation usually produced dramatic improvement in one to three sessions, augmented by a single immediate follow-up and other follow-ups every few months. In the case of patients whose physical complaints have their roots in emotional distress, I believe a health plan that includes this therapy could save a great deal of money by avoiding futile tests and surgeries.

The anxiety of repressed feelings provokes deep anguish and somatic symptoms such as muscular and skeletal pain, headaches, and irritable bowel syndrome, and these symptoms produce more anxiety. A visit to a doctor who takes time for compassionate listening would likely be helpful. However, if the doctor orders an MRI, CT scan, or other tests and drugs, the patient will not likely suffer harm, but more than likely will not get the issue causing these physical symptoms in the first place. I found PSC sessions to expedite the process of discovering what lay beneath the symptoms and found much success for patients with these sessions. (To see an example of how a Profile Self-Confrontation is conducted, see Appendix B.)

For thirty-five years, PSC formed the centerpiece of my psychotherapy program at Scott & White. It proved a powerful tool for cutting through the natural resistance all of us use to protect ourselves from our most disturbing thoughts. With both inpatients and outpatients Profile Self-Confrontation allowed me to reach the breakthroughs in diagnosis and treatment in days instead of requiring weeks, months, or even years.

Epilogue

I know that repressed emotions are the cause of most disabling illnesses. Because of this, I listened until I really heard, and it became easy for me to discover the real cause of the symptoms. I could also limit the amount of medicine and procedures that were expensive, too often ineffective, and sometimes dangerous. Before sophisticated diagnostic equipment was developed, physicians had to listen. Questions I asked repeatedly were, "Tell me how long you've had this problem. What was going on with you at that time? How did this happen? Tell me about it. What does your problem keep you from doing? What's been going on? Tell me more about it. What have other doctors told you? Was that helpful? What does your spouse or partner think about it? What medicines are you taking? What medicines did your doctor prescribe? How much are you actually taking? How can anyone possibly understand the problems you are stuck with?"

I asked enough questions to get my patients started, and then I listened. My driving force was listening, and compassion was my greatest tool. I had an amazing, rewarding career, filled with "flow" experiences. I was never satisfied with making a snap decision and prescribing a pill, and I felt like I made a difference in peoples' lives.

All of us can and should maximize our energy for living, for doing the work that will provide us with a good measure of bliss, security, and intimacy and a life filled with loving relationships, and ultimately allow us to die with a feeling of a life well-lived. But it always requires taking risks. My mentor liked to tell the story of his five-year-old daughter, who was jealous of her older brothers' ability to ride bicycles without training wheels. She was determined to compete with them. Her father could not bear watching her fall over again and again, so he retired to his study. When she finally came in, she was covered with scrapes and bruises but was squealing with delight, "I did it, I did it."

Howard looked up at her as she continued. "You ride and you fall off, you ride and you fall off, you ride and you fall off. Then you ride and you ride." My patients who learned to manage their lives by examining their dreams, meditating, painting, writing, exercising, and eating well seemed to have enough energy and self-confidence to take risks and begin to eliminate the forces that held them back. They seemed to allow themselves a "wonderment fix" by examining the world of beauty around them. They learned to "ride."

My goal, when I was practicing psychiatry, was to help my patients gain a deeper understanding of their problems and to look for the underlying causes of their symptoms. The medical institution at that time had supported my goal. At the end of my career my goal was to make sure the medical residents learned effective techniques to get to the underlying causes of their patients' complaints. But I soon realized that major changes were under way in the practice of psychiatry all across the country..

Most residents presented their patients in the way all psychiatric departments now mandated. They would spend a short time with the patient and take a brief history so they could make a diagnosis and establish a treatment plan. This was often only a prescription for medicine. Seldom did the residents ask about the underlying causes of their patients' problems during this initial diagnostic visit.

I did not give up easily, but finally, after five years, I decided to stop supervising and spend more time in my sculpture garden. For me, finding the sculpture in the marble was more satisfying than trying to change the psychiatric system.

Nevertheless, I couldn't get the change in psychiatry from listening to prescriptions off my mind. I knew the same kind of patients I had seen were, and continued to be, desperately seeking help. I continued supervising the psychiatric residents for another five years. One day while chiseling away on a marble block, I realized that until I wrote down my experiences to share with others, I wouldn't be able to stop grieving over the changes that had occurred. After thirty-four years of empathetic and active listening to patients and teaching medical school students and residents, I retired from Scott & White Clinic in Temple, Texas, to become a full-time sculptor and a part-time psychiatrist.

Some days, as I chip away at the marble, I dare to hope that listening may well regain recognition as one of the most valuable skills for all care-givers.

Appendix A
Relived Emotional Assessment Guide
Developed by Paul Ekman, Ph.D.

NAME:_____

DATE: _____

This work is focused on helping you feel several different emotional states. You will be asked to recall and relive emotions that you felt during a past event in your life and to repeat an emotional statement a few times with suggestions to help you intensify these feelings. As you say the emotional phrases, convey the feeling with your face, voice, and body. Do you have any questions? Rest and empty your mind of all thoughts, feelings, and memories. (Wait fifteen seconds)

The first emotion you are to feel is happiness. I want you to remember a time in your life when you experienced a strong feeling of happiness and when you felt pleasure in your life and activities. Tell me about that time. Now go back into that time and try to feel the happiness that you felt then. When you begin to feel the happiness again, let the feeling grow, and when you are feeling the happiness as strongly as you can, say "I feel happy." (Pause for reply) Say, "I feel happy," again with even more feeling. (Pause for reply)

Gather in all the happiness you have ever experienced and show it in your face, voice and body until you are feeling hqappiness as strongly as you can. Once again repeat, "I feel happy!" with as much emotion as you can. Now rest. (Wait fifteen seconds)

Suppose number one represents no feelings of happiness, and number eight represents the most happiness you have ever felt in your life. How much happiness did you feel just now?

Write down the number: _____

Did you feel the most happiness the first, second or third time

143

you said, "I feel happy."

Write down the number_____
Did you feel any other emotion when you were saying, "I feel happy." Write down the number _____ (If the response is negative, quickly run through the list. Did you feel any surprise ___, anger ___, disgust,___, sadness ___?) Fill in blanks with a number representing depth of feeling.

Now we will take a brief break and then move on to the next emotion. There are seven emotions to be explored in this manner. They are:
Happiness
Contempt
Fear
Anger
Disgust
Sadness
Relief

Appendix B
Profile Self-Confrontation Session

The following illustrates how a Profile Self-Confrontation session is conducted and includes dialogue with one patient.

In October 2006 I was invited to give a Psychiatric Grand Rounds, a monthly educational session, at The University of Texas Medical Branch. I met with the multimedia team, and we quickly set up a Profile Self-Confrontation arrangement: two video cameras, a monitor, and a split-screen device. I began by showing some of my tapes of Profile Self-Confrontation interviews that demonstrated how rapidly patients obtained insight into their internal conflicts and also how dramatically the face was transformed from looking sick to looking well.

After my initial remarks, I asked if one of the students would help me demonstrate the techniques I used. Immediately a handsome young man raised his right arm as he stood up saying, "I will!" He was surrounded by a bevy of attractive female medical students who smiled at him approvingly as he strode down to the front of the lecture hall. The session went like the following:

RR: What's your name?
Robert: Ebeling. Robert Ebeling.
RR: All right, Robert, I want you to sit in the green chair.
Robert: The green chair? (The audience laughed.)
RR (to the technician): Bring the camera down so both sides are level, nose to nose.
Robert: Did I part my hair straight? (The audience laughed again. Robert was clearly popular with his classmates.)
RR: Keep your head straight. (Robert looked up at the large monitor, where his right profile faced his left profile.)
Robert: That's more of me than I've ever seen.
RR: Okay, Robert, put your finger on your left cheek.
Robert: Okay. On the left side? (Somewhat hesitantly, Robert touched the left side of his face.)
RR: Yup. That's your left side. (The audience laughed.)

145

RR: Can the audience hear? (They responded with a chorus of "yes.")

RR: I want you to make a lot of faces, Robert. Stick out your tongue, open and close your eyes, go a little faster. (Robert blinked his eyes, stuck out his tongue, crunched up his face.)

RR: How does that feel?

Robert: Pretty good.

RR: Take a look at your left profile. Do you see any difference in your profiles?

Robert: Yeah, my left side looks lighter. It looks more cautious than the right side.

RR: "Cautious."

Robert: I guess. If I had to go with one, I guess I'd go with two of my right sides.

RR: Now, is your right side the one you show to the world?

Robert: I would hope so. (Both he and the audience laughed.) That seems to be the more confident one.

RR: Can you name one of them, Robert?

Robert: I could, I guess. (The audience chuckled.)

RR: That's what I want you to do.

Robert: I'll name any name, or thing, or person?

RR: Yeah.

Robert: I'll name the right side Robert.

RR (pointing to the right side of Robert's face): Is he Robert?

Robert: I would think so. He looks more like me.

RR: Then the other side. What's his name?

Robert: Oh, I think Joe probably comes out when people bring out your shortcomings, and you have to—pretty much everything you do in medical school is wrong. So I've been seeing a lot of Joe lately. (The audience laughed knowingly.)

RR: Have you ever been on good terms with Joe?

Robert: Sure.

RR: When was that?

Robert: It's been a while.

RR: Are you making fun of Joe?

Robert: No, I'm not making fun of Joe, but I think if it were up to Robert, he would be perfect and never need criticism.

RR: Yes. Did you notice your voice went up?

Robert: Sorry. No, I didn't know that.

RR: That means you are being defensive.

Robert: Does that mean I'm being defensive of Joe?

RR: Umhum.

Robert: Okay.

RR: Tell me more about Joe.

Robert: I think . . .

RR: Your voice went way up.

Robert: I think when we talk about Joe, he accepts criticism a little more internally. He lets it get to him more than Robert.

RR: Is Joe an introvert?

Robert: Yes, sir!

RR: Does Joe write poetry?

Robert: He could try. He did at one time.

RR: When was that?

Robert: In college.

RR: And then you followed the medical track.

Robert: Yes. He was—Joe was, and also Robert was—a philosophy major before.

RR: What did Joe think about you going into medical school?

Robert: Joe liked it, but he probably wasn't too comfortable with so many levels above him. No one is lower on the totem pole than a third-year medical student.

RR: Whose idea was it to go to med school?

Robert: Probably Robert's.

RR: And where did he get that idea?

Robert: Well . . .

RR: Was your father a doctor?

Robert: Yes, he is.

RR: What do you think about that? (Robert didn't answer.)

RR: Well, my father is a doctor. It kind of goes around.

Robert: I guess so.

RR: How are you feeling right now?

Robert: I don't know, little anxious, a little nervous.

RR: You're on stage.

Robert: Yeah, I know. I've never seen a six-foot me, my face being six feet, anyway.

RR: So Robert had to be a doctor? I know something about that.

Robert: He expected himself to be.

RR: Are you the oldest child?

Robert: Yes.

RR: What does that mean?

Robert: More strict, more leeway?

RR: What were your parents' expectations like? (Robert shrugged.)

RR: What's your dad's first name?

Robert: Robert. I'm the third.

RR: What about your mother? Does she like Joe or does she like Robert?

Robert: She likes them both.

RR: What just came to your mind?

Robert: The decision between . . . my parents.

RR: Yes.

Robert: They were pretty much okay with me going to medical school or not. I never felt pushed to go one way or another.

RR: So Robert's going to be a psychiatrist?

Robert: Is he?

RR: Yeah.

Robert: It would be better than OB/GYN. (The audience laughed as if responding to an inside joke.) At this point in the interview, Robert became aware of the significant conflict between his profiles. The unrecognized, feeling side, Joe, the poet and philosopher, was right there for all to see.

RR: Why are you being so defensive?

Robert: Probably because it's true.

RR: You're smiling.

Robert: I'm sure, absolutely. It's just that I think that I can't let anyone see how I'm really feeling, how Joe feels.

RR: Could Robert let Joe express himself?

Robert: He never has.

RR: Really?

Robert: Yes.

148

RR: Every person has a god and devil in him. The conflict takes so much energy.

Robert: I think there's always going to be conflict—even within yourself.

RR: Big conflict. How do you feel about that?

Robert: Sometimes Joe has to take in the information and process it in a way that's acceptable to Robert.

RR: I want to do an emotional status exam now.

Robert: Okay.

RR: Go back to a time when you were angry, so angry that you wanted to hit someone or did hit someone. Have you ever felt that way?

Robert: Absolutely.

RR: Are you looking angry?

Robert: What am I supposed to say?

RR: Robert smiles when he's angry, which invites more anger.

Robert: I don't think he invites more anger, just that he is angrier.

RR: Look at your face! What mask are you hiding behind?

Robert: From myself or from others?

RR: What kind of mask are you wearing?

Robert: I always thought you were your own worst enemy.

RR: Let's try another emotion. Disgust. (Robert's nose immediately wrinkled.)

RR: There's your snout reflex. You have no trouble with disgust. (Robert spontaneously wrinkled his nose again.)

RR: There it is again. When you see someone wrinkle his nose you know he is experiencing disgust. Now, let's look at sad, a time when you were very, very sad. Can you remember a time like that?

Robert: Yeah, I can.

RR: Look at yourself. What are you doing?

Robert: Probably my mouth is relaxing. My eyes get a little bigger.

RR: Probably?

Robert: That probably I should qualify everything, that noth-

149

ing is black and white.

RR: We now know you have trouble with sadness and anger. Is it helpful for you to know that?

Robert: Yes.

RR: If you can't express anger, then people will continue to make you angry and that's valuable to know. If Robert lets Joe get more involved, you won't see so much smiling. At the end of the interview, the room was silent. Robert and the audience were aware that he had begun psychotherapy. I then pointed out to the audience that the nonverbal stuff is where a therapist and patient have to go, like facial expressions and body language. When I notice a patient's voice is way up, I know I am probably not making any progress. Profile Self-Confrontation, like poetry, painting, music, and dreams, for me, was an excellent way to cut corners and rapidly get to deep feelings. These methods sliced through the intellect and quickly got to the emotions because what patients painted or wrote or saw on a screen was right in front of them. One year after the Grand Rounds, I received this letter from Robert. He asked me to use his real name.

Dear Dr. Rynearson,

The experience as a whole was quite amazing. I am not one to believe in things that do not have a documented study to prove them, so I was greatly skeptical about the entire process. Perhaps it was my need to see it for myself, or maybe it was just Joe coming out to play; either way I raised my hand and volunteered to have the two sides of my face blown up to eight feet by six feet on the stage. Then things became a little more serious.

I remember sitting in the chair looking at the two sides of my face thinking, "Are those both me?" I was asked then to name the two sides of my face. This was a little awkward as I knew it was my face, but at the same time they did look different. The right side of my face I remember looking more stoic, more objective, and since that was how I try to project myself, I named that side "Robert." The left side was decidedly more personable, more emotional; he even had a slight smile on his face! That side I called "Joe." We then talked frankly about the two sides of my face, how they were different and what they said about me.

I told you that all my life I have tried to be objective in all that I do. I thought that my friends could count on me to give them an honest opinion, that they could trust me. I myself hate when emotion takes control of a situation, especially one of life and death, which I will face as a physician, so I strived to take it out of my equation. The right side of my face mirrored closely what I had tried to become, hence the name, "Robert." The left side of my face was the side I actually did not like. It seemed more emotional, more apt to whimsy, but at the same time it actually looked happy. I named this side "Joe" after a friend of mine who always took things lightly and never let me take myself too seriously. He was a great friend. Then we discussed why the two sides of my face were so different, and they were. After some searching we came to the conclusion that I was indeed taking myself too seriously and that I needed to lighten up occasionally. I needed to let "Joe" play a little. It definitely would make life a little brighter, and I could still be objective with a smile on my face.

So what started as a curious volunteering ended up altering my life. I have taken your advice, and my own, to take life a little lighter and definitely not to take myself too seriously. The change has impacted my relationship with my then girlfriend, now wife, the most. I am now thought of as a serious, yet happy person who will take the time to smell the roses of life and not stomp on the past with the pretense that I am purely objective and emotionless.

Thank you again, Dr. Rynearson

Appendix C

This is the letter I received from Lauren, a patient at Scott & White Clinic, who asked that her real name be withheld:

Growing up, I was often called "the curly haired, kindest girl with the beautiful, innocent eyes." I was the first person to invite a new person to "sit by me" or come over for a visit. I made perfect grades without studying. Also, I was the girl who screamed at my mother when trying on clothes, the girl who told the first dirty joke at a sixth-grade party, and the girl who invited my seventh grade teacher to "Go to Hell!" to get attention in front of the whole class (and ruin my mother's plans for the afternoon).

I quickly learned, however, how to hide this demonic side in order to sustain an empathic, nurturing, and high-achieving persona because the rewards of social and academic success gave immediate satisfaction. I just repressed my cynical thoughts about the "joke" that most institutions appeared to be—pretty uncomfortable when it came to religion and education.

This pattern continued throughout most of my adult life, and with the "saving grace" being that my husband, who has been my boyfriend since ninth grade, knew and shared this talent for seeing through or into the appearance of the world around him.

One of the reasons I fell so in love with him, in retrospect, was that I could safely share my insights with him as he could with me in our private world of analysis! My graduate level study of literature also gave me the vicarious outlet of the "oft thought, but ne'er so well expressed."

In my profession as a teacher, most of my students would see me as smart and kind, staying up hours to write recommendations or tutor reluctant learners. I can "bring together" a class to feel as one when studying novels, stories, essays, and poems which deal with the universal human suffering—Matthew Arnold's "Eternal Note of Sadness." I can also lay into a student who is persistently irresponsible or inconsiderate and can take pride at times in the statement, "A lot of people are afraid of you."

As a parent, however, I had a difficult time reconciling with my nurturing side. I was "fun" to be around, we read together, we traveled, we sang and danced together with abandon, and I created ways that my children could feel good about themselves when befriending an "outsider."

I was also manipulative and impatient, making them practice the piano, read aloud, hurry through bath time, or yelling at persistent behavior I could not control. I tried to "make" them reflective and introverted but also sociable and popular.

Ever since studying Freud and Jung, and so many others, I have been able to intellectually "own" my "shadow side" as an inevitable part of a healthy personality. Emotionally, however, the guilt and then the anger associated with thispart of me have been too painful to ignore.

The profile study I asked Dr. Rynearson to do with me was an incomparable avenue for helping those two sides of me "dialogue" with each other with specific instances from my life and, finally, to incorporate and celebrate this seeming dichotomy as one person.

I still have "talks" with myself when I am tempted to oversimplify others or me as "good" or "bad," and have used this duality as an important tool in teaching character analysis so that students can more readily identify with the complexity of the human psyche.

Thank you for getting my selves together.

Lauren

Works Cited

Becker, Ernest. *The Denial of Death.* Detroit: Free P, 1997.

Carroll, Lewis. *Alice in Wonderland.* Los Angeles: Hallmark, 1999

Craik, Dinah Mulock. *A Life for a Life.* Leipzig: Tauchnitz, 1859. Montana: Kessinger, 2004.

Doidge, Norman, MD. *The Brain That Changes Itself.* New York: Penguin, 2007.

Durant, Will. *The Story of Civilization.* Vol. 7. New York: Simon, 1961.

Eckstein, Gustav. *The Body Has a Head.* New York: Harper, 1970

Edel, Leon. "The Madness of Art." *The American Journal of Psychiatry* 32 (1975): 1005-1012.

Gilbert, Daniel. *Stumbling on Happiness.* New York: Knopf, 2006.

Menninger, Karl A., MD. "Polysurgery and Polysurgical Addiction." *Psychoanalytic Quarterly* 3 (1034): 173-199.

Osler, William. *The Principles and Practice of Medicine.* New York: Appleton, 1925.

Percy, Walker. *Lost in the Cosmos.* New York: Picador, 2000.

Wolff, Werner. *Expression of Personality.* New York: Harper, 1943

Yalom, Irvin, MD. *Existential Psychotherapy.* New York: Basic Books, 1980

Suggestions for Discussion

1. Which of Walker Percy's choices would you select to describe yourself?
   A. Positive
   B. Negative
   C. Neither A nor B
   D. Both A and B

2. Have you ever noticed differences in your own profile?

3. Why do actors insist photos be taken of their "good" side?

4. If you put two of your right profiles together to make a whole face and two left profiles together to make a whole face, what would you look like? You can do this on your computer by reversing the photo, cutting, and pasting.

5. Have you ever had a prophetic dream?

6. What have you learned about yourself from looking at old family photographs?

7. Has anyone ever helped you to gain enough insight to have an "Aha!" moment?

8. What does the old saying "Apples don't fall far from the tree" mean?

9. When was the first time you risked running to second base without taking first base with you?

10. When was the last time you took such a risk?

11. William James said, "Feelings follow action." What does that mean?

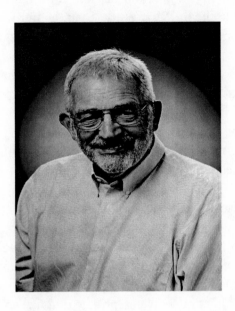

ABOUT THE AUTHOR

The son of a Mayo Clinic endocrinologist and an artist mother, Bob Rynearson was born in Rochester, Minnesota, in 1932. After graduating from Harvard with a bachelor's degree in liberal arts, he attended the University of Minnesota School of Medicine.

Throughout his academic career, he maintained a strong interest in art, spending much of his spare time sculpting. In 1962, he completed his psychiatric residency at the Mayo Foundation. He then served as assistant medical director at the Rochester State Hospital until moving to Temple, Texas, in 1965 to establish the Department of Psychiatry at Scott & White Clinic, a multi-specialty clinic modeled after Mayo.

When Texas A&M University established its medical school in 1978, Dr. Rynearson became the first chairman of its Department of Psychiatry, a position he held until his retirement from academic medicine in 1997. While chair, he introduced numerous innovative concepts in inpatient and outpatient psychotherapy, including the use of art and videography.

He and his wife, Marjie, built a house that accommodated their passions for studio art and provided an environment for encouraging similar interests in their four sons.

The compound grew to include studios for silk-screening, ceramics, paper-making, sculpting, and glass-blowing. For inspiration, Dr. Rynearson traveled to Alaska and to the Sepik River in Papuau, New Guinea, where he studied totem poles and masks.

He was fascinated by how indigenous artists captured emotion in their depictions of human faces. He applied these insights and techniques to his own sculpture in wood, marble, and clay and also to a technique called Profile Self-Confrontation, a shortcut to the unconscious.

He divides his time between private practice and sculpting. He is an emeritus Fellow of the American Psychiatric Association, the American College of Psychiatry and the Southern Psychiatric Association, of which he is past president.

LaVergne, TN USA
09 June 2010
185507LV00003B/5/P